SEARCHING FOR THE OPEN DOOR
A WOMAN'S STRUGGLE FOR SURVIVAL
AFTER A TRAUMATIC BRAIN INJURY

Cynthia Paddock Doroghazi

New River Publications, LLC   Ft. Lauderdale, FL

To Barb and Bruce —
Many thanks for your patronage.
May you have fun on your new trike!
Warm regards,
Cynthia Doroghazi

Published by New River Publications
2860 SR 84
Suite 116, PMB 202
Ft. Lauderdale, FL 33312
(954) 636-1936
www.newriverpublications.com

Printed in the United States of America
LCCN: 2007932982

Doroghazi, Cynthia P.
ISBN 9780979822711

Cover design by Mark Riddle

This book is dedicated to all my friends and family who supported me throughout this terrible ordeal, who were instrumental in my recovery, and who kept saying to me, "You really need to write a book about this."

Most especially,
To my mother, Blair Alexander Paddock, and to the memory of my father, Robert Bradford Paddock, Esq. (1920-1999) and to my husband, Stephen Robert Doroghazi, Esq. all of whom have exemplified and personified the true meaning of love in my life

WHAT PEOPLE ARE SAYING ABOUT THIS BOOK

This is a nearly destroyed woman's riveting, page-turning story of re-creation out of chaos and darkness, a near-mythic struggle with the nearly invincible forces of the medical and insurance establishment. The author experiences re-generation, not overnight, but one breath, one step, one day at a time. Angels in the guise of mortals appear to walk with her through the valley of the shadow of death and, what's worse, legal proceedings. Through it all she discovers that life is hard—sometimes impossibly hard—but grace abounds. Behold, life is good. Not perfect. But pretty darn good, after all.

> DR. RANDALL TREMBA, PASTOR
> SHEPHERDSTOWN PRESBYTERIAN CHURCH
> EXECUTIVE EDITOR
> THE GOOD SHEPHERD/GOOD NEWS PAPER
> SHEPHERDSTOWN, WEST VIRGINIA

After years of struggle, Cynthia finally completed her master's degree at SAIS. At the graduation, her classmates gave her a standing ovation. After you read this book, you will understand why they did. Cynthia's story is an inspirational demonstration of what courage, determination and sheer willpower can accomplish in the face of seemingly life-destroying injuries. There is a message here for the families and care-givers of other victims of traumatic brain injury – don't underestimate what can be accomplished with will and support. And for those of us fortunate not to have suffered what Cynthia has, the message is to be grateful for our good fortune and to work as hard as Cynthia has to make use of the abilities we have been given.

> PAUL WOLFOWITZ, FORMER DEAN, 1994-2001
> THE JOHNS HOPKINS UNIVERSITY
> SCHOOL OF ADVANCED INTERNATIONAL STUDIES

All of us face challenges and barriers in life. We are only as big as the smallest thing it takes to divert us from our calling. Through Cynthia's struggles, we can all learn how to move toward our own destiny.

> JIM STOVALL, AUTHOR OF <u>THE ULTIMATE GIFT</u>

Searching for the Open Door exposes the dirty little secrets of medical malpractice. Cynthia Paddock Doroghazi lets the malpractice victim know what to expect in a lawsuit and she lets malpractice lawyers know what their clients are thinking. She has lived the tale and boldly provides insight into the behind-the-scene process of a modern day malpractice lawsuit. She demonstrates, without a lot of legal jargon, the need to preserve the American common law malpractice lawsuit system.

"A winner. Long live the pursuit of justice!"

> JACK H. OLENDER
> THE MALPRACTICE LAW FIRM
> OF JACK H. OLENDER AND ASSOCIATES, P.C.
> WASHINGTON, D. C.

John Lennon once wrote, "The price of anything is the amount of life you exchange for it". On one level, then, this book is priceless...priceless for the toll that Ms. Paddock's brain injury extracted from her. On the other hand, this book would never have been written without that expense. And as a clinician that has become all too familiar with the tragedy of traumatic brain injury (TBI), it is an absolute delight to see someone of Ms. Paddock's character rise above it all to pass on a message of hope and inspiration. There *is* life after a TBI and in reading her account of the long road back, I couldn't put the book down.

> TERRY G. SHAW, PH.D., ABPN
> CHIEF NEUROPSYCHOLOGIST
> COMPREHENSIVE COMMUNITY
> REHABILITATION SERVICES

This book will be a great inspiration to anyone who has been dealt a raw hand by life, by showing them what faith and perseverance can accomplish. It is also a gripping story of one young woman's struggle with a big and impersonal medical bureaucracy that can destroy lives as well as save them.

> FRANCIS FUKUYAMA
> DIRECTOR, INTERNATIONAL DEVELOPMENT
> THE JOHNS HOPKINS UNIVERSITY
> SCHOOL OF ADVANCED INTERNATIONAL STUDIES

When I began to read **Searching for the Open Door** by Cynthia Paddock Doroghazi, I could not put the book down! I thought I would quickly flip through the pages, learn a little bit and get back to work. But I was so impressed with the way the author led me through the search that I had to read on.

Cynthia is a walking miracle, and an amazing example of how proper medical care can play a part in one's recovery. Her book sends a strong message to all of our doctors, nurses and therapists, reminding them how much the work they do every day makes an impact on people's lives.

Medical professionals alone cannot heal a person. It takes a unique combination of the right treatment, at the right time, from the right place, to a willing patient, along with blessings from above. Cynthia was lucky to have all of these things, working together, to help her recover from this tragic injury.

I encourage you to take the journey that **Searching for the Open Door** offers. You will be captivated, amazed, humbled, and gain a new appreciation for how precious every day is. Nobody is promised tomorrow, but we can certainly follow our author's lead, and live each and every day with a smile!

> MARK CHILUTTI
> ASSISTANT VICE-PRESIDENT - DEVELOPMENT
> MAGEE REHAB HOSPITAL FOUNDATION
> PHILADELPHIA, PENNSYLVANIA

This is a moving and inspiring story of what courage, faith and hard work can accomplish.

> MICHAEL MANDELBAUM
> PROFESSOR OF AMERICAN FOREIGN POLICY
> THE JOHNS HOPKINS UNIVERSITY
> SCHOOL OF ADVANCED INTERNATIONAL STUDIES

When one door of happiness closes, another opens; but often we look so long at the closed door that we do not see the one which has opened for us.

Helen Keller

"When God wounds from on high, he will follow with the remedy."

Fernando de Rojas (c.1465-c.1538)
in La Celestina

TABLE OF CONTENTS

ACKNOWLEDGEMENTS

First and foremost, I would like to thank the many physical therapists, occupational therapists and speech therapists who brought me back to life and without whom I could not have written this book. I would not be the woman I am today without each and every one of them.

At The George Washington University Medical Center in Washington, D. C., they include Julie Ries, my physical therapist, Ann Whitzig and Daphne Stanza, my speech therapists and Susan Hannah Phantom, my occupational therapist.

At Magee Rehabilitation Hospital in Philadelphia, Pennsylvania, I would like to thank Lawrence J. Horn, M.D., the attending physiatrist, Jayne Weinstock, my speech therapist, Janet Standview and Teresa Vaccaro, my physical therapists, and Janet Rohlender, Kathy Maley, and Sharon Beyer, my occupational therapists. I will always be grateful to Colleen Salemo, who was my primary day nurse at Magee and the only one brave enough to put in my contact lenses and to Carmen Kiernan, who gave me a whole new perspective on bathing and whose endless patience was a credit to her character.

At PATE Rehabilitation Endeavors, Inc. in Dallas Texas, I cannot express enough gratitude to my principal therapist, Barbara Hingom, whose patience and willingness to work with me despite my frequent temper tantrums and in spite of my ungrateful attitude was exemplary. Lisa Protsman and Jeanne Sowers were my physical therapists, and Donna P. Thomas was my occupational therapist.

At Hillcrest's Kaiser Rehabilitation program in Tulsa, Oklahoma, I would like to thank Janis E. Lambdin, my speech therapist, Terry Henshaw and Carol Wycoff, my physical therapists, David Coffman and Sue Wilkinson, my occupational therapists, and Terry Shaw, the neuropsychologist whose fatherly advice has become my mantra.

I would never have found these latter two rehabilitation venues if it had not been for the efforts of two case workers hired by Blue Cross/Blue Shield of Maryland. Those caseworkers were Linda Cosby, in Washington and Claire Guiseffi, RN in Dallas.

There are many people who have helped me return to some semblance of a normal life upon my return to The Johns Hopkins School of Advanced International Studies (SAIS). They include the late George L. Crowell, the Associate Dean of Students at SAIS while I was a student there, Betty Beauchamp, the Registrar during my time at SAIS and Priscilla Fruchtar, the Director of Financial Aid. Francis Fukuyama, the Director of the International Development program and the Bernard Schwartz Professor of International Political Economy, and Paul Wolfowitz, the Dean of SAIS when I graduated and while I was on the staff there, both helped make my transition into the working world a little easier. In addition, I wish to thank Michael Mandelbaum, the Christian A. Herter Professor of American Foreign Policy and the director of the American Foreign Policy program and his wife, Anne Mandelbaum, a professional writer, editor, and photographer, who is also an attorney. Both were unwavering in their support, not only of me, but also of my mother and father, during the ordeal of my injury and recovery, and to this day.

I will always be grateful to Sam Shriver, the insurance representative for the school, who made further rehabilitation possible and to Susan Ryerson, my physical therapist in Washington, D. C., whose innovative approaches and sensitivity make her a credit to her profession.

I would also like to thank the many friends, who helped make my transition back into school an easier one and who visited me every day while I was in the hospital for the original surgery and for subsequent ones. In particular, I would like to thank the following: Sylvie Bossoutrot, Eric Brody, Burke Burnett, Robert Dudley, Maria Gracheva, Bruce Hammond, Geoffrey Haskell, Brin Luther, Paul Marin, David Skarinsky, Erick White, Laurie Winslow, and James Wood.

Both friends and family played an enormous role in my recovery and in preparing this book for publication. I would like to give special thanks to my two sisters, Susan and Carolyn Paddock, who took turns editing portions of the manuscript. Pat Perfetto proofread the entire manuscript. Francis Fukuyama, my supervisor when I worked at SAIS, John Schidlovsky, the Director of the International Reporting Project at SAIS and Anne and Michael Mandelbaum read through parts of my manuscript and the book proposal and provided suggestions, great encouragement and great advice along the way.

I would also like to thank Jack H. Olender, Marian K. Riedy, and the late Gary S. Freeman for their care in prosecuting my case. Without their efforts, I would not be able to enjoy the life I have now. Marian, in particular, who was the assisting attorney on my case, was instrumental in helping me reconstruct the trial. She edited that portion of the book.

Last but not least, I am very grateful to my husband, Steve, who gave me the courage and support I needed to finally put pen to paper. He spent many hours editing the entire manuscript and then reading through it several times in its various forms.

Foreword

On one April morning in 1994, Cynthia Paddock walked into my physical therapy clinic. Her balance was precarious, her walk was slow with a noticeable limp, and she juggled a bag and a purse on one shoulder while struggling with her cane in her right hand. Sitting down, she looked around and, staring straight at me, said, "Everyone tells me I should be content with how I am now, that I will not get any more recovery, and that I will always have to wear this ugly brace. I refuse to believe this is as good as it gets." She began to cry.

Over the course of the eleven years I treated her, Cynthia and I developed trust and formed a bond. She confided in me her worries, which ran from the immediate to the long term: "I can't walk to the bathroom at night. I can't walk across the city street. I can't wear regular shoes. I don't have enough energy to work. How will I support myself? How will I be able to really live alone?" I dealt with her immediate concern, that the brace was large, bulky and caused sores on her foot, and reassured her that we would make a smaller brace that would allow her to wear regular shoes. I also gave her hope that, someday, she might be able to walk with greater ease.

In some ways, Cynthia resembled my other clients. New clients, who come to my practice, have usually finished their intensive physical rehabilitation and have one thing in common. They are determined to continue to recover despite the medical practitioners' claims that the recovery window is only two years. But Cynthia had something more. She had a determination to return to a life that she could accept.

Recovery from a brain injury requires more than good medical and rehabilitative care, courage and a willingness to work hard. It requires a determination to return to an acceptable life. And a therapist must always hold out the hope for a return to this acceptable life; a life where one's former underlying strengths and passions are adapted to new realities. Physical therapy, for people such as Cynthia, is not merely a technical exercise; it is also aimed at psychological recovery – restoring the hope for a meaningful life.

For Cynthia, this recovery began with her challenge to me to help her walk with more dignity. Over the next eleven years, I witnessed her life as it went from one of despair to one in which she had a fulfilling professional life, fell in love and got married. In writing this book, I know she has achieved one of her long-term goals. I expect that she will achieve many more goals over her lifetime, because I suspect that Cynthia's recovery has not ended.

Susan Ryerson, PT, ScD

Preface

This book is about my physical, emotional and spiritual reawakening after what I was told by an eminent neurosurgeon would be a routine surgery on May 7, 1990. That surgery left me in a three-week coma, a three-month long semi-vegetative state, and completely paralyzed on the left side of my body.

This is a story of hope and the triumph of the human spirit over what seemed to be insurmountable odds. It is a story about the struggle to survive against all odds, and about the support of family and friends. More significantly, it is about accepting the loss of previous dreams and plans and finding a new sense of purpose for living that, although unexpected and, in a sense, undesired, nevertheless becomes something greater than what could ever have been imagined.

I hope that this book will appeal to a wide range of people: people who feel lost, overwhelmed by the cards they've been dealt and need a reason to keep going; people who feel hopeless about their situations and the course that their life has taken; people who are confronted with a devastating physical illness such as cancer or multiple sclerosis, or any other illnesses, both physical and psychological; people who are frustrated with fighting against the inflexibility and medical ignorance of insurance company representatives, and other large, impersonal bureaucracies. Finally, I hope this book will appeal to people who can appreciate the power of love, prayer, friendship, and family ties, even if they, themselves, have never experienced these blessings.

1

The Traumatic Brain Injury

I hear voices and the sounds of traffic, cars honking. I'm dimly aware of being strapped onto a stretcher. I cannot move anything but my head. I call out. "Where am I? How did I get here? What happened? What's going on? Where am I going?" These are the questions flooding my mind. I hear voices. They try to calm me down, talking to me in a soothing tone of voice. "You are in an ambulance, being transported to Philadelphia." "Don't worry," they say. "Your parents are right behind us." It is August 13, 1990. I am twenty-six years old. And this is my first conscious thought in more than three months.

*　　　　*　　　　*　　　　*

"Order in the court. Order in the court. All rise. The honorable Judge Joan Zeldon presiding." Ah, at last. April 3, 1995. I had been waiting for this day for almost five years. The day of reckoning. After five years of being in complete darkness, I will finally find out what happened to me on May 7, 1990 and how a woman undergoing a routine brain operation ended up in a coma for three weeks, in a semi-vegetative state for approximately three months and paralyzed on the entire left side of her body.

Some of the blanks I could fill in myself. I was in my second semester as a candidate for a master's degree at The Johns Hopkins University School of Advanced International Studies (SAIS) in Washington, D. C. when I began suffering from headaches. I was not overly concerned about them. After all, I was enrolled in a stressful program at a high-powered school; headaches come with the territory. However, a loud rushing sound – as when you put a shell up to your ear – began to develop in my right ear. I decided I should see a doctor. I was referred by a Tulsa-based ear, nose and throat doctor (ENT) to a neurosurgeon based in Washington, D. C., because I was living and going to school in Washington at the time. That neurosurgeon's practice was located at The George Washington University Medical Center in Washington. The surgeon's name was Dr. Edward Laws and he was said to be one of the best neurosurgeons in the country. After describing my symptoms to him, he recommended I undergo an MRI.

This was in February 1990. Dr. Laws called me a few weeks after my brain scan. His loud, cheery voice exclaimed: "Good news!" It was not a tumor in the ear canal as he had originally thought. I had a condition known as hydrocephalus, commonly known as water on the brain. The procedure used to correct this condition, he explained, is routine. All that was required was to insert a tube, a shunt, into the meninges surrounding the brain and drain off the cerebral spinal fluid (CSF) that was currently blocked and thus building up inside my head, pushing the sides of my brain against my skull. This, he explained, was what was causing the rushing sound in my ear and the headaches. So, that was that. Simple. Routine. I would be in and out of the hospital in four days, with a recovery period of two weeks. He saw no problem in my going on the internship in London for which I had just been selected, marketing voicemail equipment to Hungarian firms. I was so happy. It was all settled then. The surgery was to take place after my last final examination. My parents would fly to Washington from their home in Tulsa for the operation and be by my side during the two-week recovery period. And then I would leave for London.

Unfortunately, life had other plans for me.

At some point during the operation, the doctor nicked a blood vessel, a recognized complication of the surgery. The bleed wasn't detected at the point it occurred because my blood pressure was kept low during the operation. So, when the doctors closed me up and brought my blood pressure up, blood began to flow from the blood vessel. This, in itself, would not have caused any problems if it had been detected in a timely fashion during my recovery.

One of the main points of contention during the trial was whether it was a slow or fast bleed. The difference was important. Our evidence showed it was a slow bleed, so symptoms of the bleed should have been detected by the nurse much earlier than they were. The defense contended that I bled very fast at the very end of my recovery period, so that I could not have had any symptoms that the nurse responsible for monitoring me should have detected earlier than she actually did.

After the operation, I was transferred from the recovery room to the Neurological Concentrated Care Unit (NCCU) and it was during my stay there that the results of the hemorrhage began to manifest themselves. As the bleed progressed, it stripped the inner lining of the skull, known as the dura, away from skull wall. The bleed then began to compress the brain, shifting the brain to the left as it enlarged. My brain began to buckle. The cortex of my brain began to cut off the flow of oxygen to my brain. By the time the nurse in charge of the NCCU, Barbara Boston, noticed the signs of increased intercranial pressure (ICP) and notified the resident on call, the bleed had filled about one-quarter of the total volume of my skull, the equivalent of eighteen ounces of blood.

As a result of this massive bleed, my brain nearly collapsed in on itself and I started to go into respiratory failure. I was twenty minutes away from death before the nurse decided she should call the resident on duty. The resident, Dr. Kelly, took twenty minutes to get to my bedside, because all he knew was that the nurse was having trouble arousing me. Upon taking one look at me, he called a code blue. "Nurse, there's a reason you can't arouse your patient, she's going into arrest!" I was rushed back into surgery, where one of the surgeons performed a procedure in which he cut away part of my skull to evacuate the blood. During *that* operation, I somehow contracted e coli meningitis, bacteria that is almost always fatal and, if not fatal, usually results in severe brain damage. How I became infected with this bacterium remains a mystery, since e coli is only found in the anal region. How in the world did a bacterium found only in the anal region end up inside my brain? How indeed?

After five more operations, in which surgeons removed a portion of my skull to evacuate the blood clot (craniotomy), inserted a tube into my ventricules to drain the spinal fluid, thereby replacing the work of the non-functioning shunt (ventriculostomy), reopened the shunt and clamped off the ventriculostomy, removed the shunt because I had developed signs that my ventricles were infected (ventriculitis), inserted another ventriculostomy tube in place of the shunt, and finally replaced the original tube that ran from inside my ventricules and emptied into my abdominal cavity (ventricular-peritoneal (VP) shunt), all within a one-month period, my brain finally decided enough was enough. I slid into a coma, moving in and out of a semi-vegetative state for approximately three months. I finally became fully cognizant three months later to find myself paralyzed on the left side of my body, with the IQ of a vegetable, in diapers, being fed through a tube, able to remember very little and facing the prospect of having to relearn what a baby learns in the first years of life, such as standing, walking, and toilet training.

2

The Courtroom Drama. (April 3, 1995)[1]

Almost three years after the calamitous brain surgery and the coma that followed it, I decided to sue the neurosurgeon and the hospital where my life-changing – indeed almost life-ending – operation took place. To prepare for the trial, I needed the experts to fill in the gaps in my memory during the three months from May 7 to August 12, 1990 that were a total blank. I also needed them to help me understand exactly what had happened to me and why, as well as how much it would affect me in terms of my physical and cognitive abilities in the pursuit of my intended career.

To have the kind of disastrous outcome I had from what was presented to me by Dr. Laws as a routine operation, there is a good chance that medical negligence played a major role. It is the responsibility of the injured party to investigate every detail of the medical procedure in order to bring a lawsuit alleging negligence. If the evidence shows that indeed someone *was* negligent, the hurt party brings a lawsuit against the party that is be-

---

[1] Because this case was settled before it went to the jury, the official transcript of the court proceedings is not available. The following facts of the case are accurate. I reconstructed trial testimony from notes taken at the trial, depositions taken before the trial and interviews of persons present at the trial. Therefore, quotation marks do not necessarily reflect verbatim testimony, but are merely utilized to distinguish between who is speaking at a specific time during the trial. Specifically, direct testimony is based on depositions and cross examinations are derived through notes taken at the trial or personal memory.

lieved to be at fault in an effort to be compensated monetarily for the pain, suffering and loss of income incurred. I consulted the Washington law firm of Jack H. Olender and Associates, P.C. and retained Gary Freeman and Marian Riedy as my attorneys. My attorneys' experts, who reviewed all the medical records, determined that it was the negligent care I had received in the Neurological Concentrated Care Unit (NCCU) after my brain surgery that rendered me in a coma and paralyzed on one side.

There are two types of lawsuits: criminal and civil. While a criminal trial is brought by the government against an individual, a civil lawsuit is brought by individuals, corporations, or partnerships against other individuals, corporations or partnerships. Instead of a prison sentence, which is often the result of a criminal defendant being found guilty, in a civil trial, the party who is found responsible for the injury, i.e. the guilty party, must pay money directly to the plaintiff, the party who was injured. Often, it is the defendant's insurance company that pays the damage award. The plaintiff presents its case first. All the witnesses called to testify on the plaintiff's behalf are known as plaintiff's witnesses. The individual or entity being sued is known as the defendant. All the witnesses called to testify on the defendant's behalf are known as defense witnesses. In my case, the defendant was The George Washington University Medical Center (GWUMC), the employer of Barbara Boston, the nurse whose inaction was most likely responsible for the extent of my traumatic brain injury. The gist of my case was that the nursing care was negligent, and the Hospital was responsible for the negligence of its employee acting within the scope of her employment. In addition, we alleged that the Hospital was *independently* negligent in failing to adequately train nurse Barbara Boston.

Many years can pass between the time that the injured party is well enough and able to file a lawsuit and the time that the case actually comes to trial. In my case, my complaint was filed on March 24, 1993, almost three years since the operation and two years before the trial actually began. In those two years, both the plaintiff and the defendant used the time to locate and depose their witnesses. The deposition is part of the process during which both sides determine all the relevant facts of the case and decide who will testify and what each witness will say. This is called the "discovery" phase of a trial. There are countless briefs or motions that each side files with the court, in which one side argues its case and lays out in detail what will be covered, the nature of the complaint, and the amount of damages that it seeks. After numerous pre-trial motions, a judge sets a trial date to hear the case.

What made *my* trial so difficult for my lawyers was the fact that, by 1993, I no longer appeared as if I had undergone a major medical ordeal. I had a small brace on my left ankle and I walked with a cane, but other than that, I did not look particularly "damaged." In fact, seeing me, one would have no idea that anything had happened to me at all or that I was entitled to any kind of monetary relief whatsoever.

As I look back at the two weeks of the trial, five major events stand out in my mind. The first was the jury selection. The make-up of the jury is always important, but it was especially crucial in my case. I was a young, thin, highly-educated Caucasian woman, who had always been considered attractive. My attorneys would be asking the jurors to "put themselves in my place," to "be my peers," in an effort to convince them to be sympathetic to my plight and, accordingly, render a large monetary award for my damages, pain, and suffering. Who from the jury pool would truly be able to put themselves in my place?

During the process of jury selection, I sat behind my attorney as the parade of jurors entered the courtroom through a door in the back. The courtroom of the Superior Court of the District of Columbia was rather plain and austere. In the front of the courtroom sat the judge on a platform with a huge desk surrounding her and microphones on top of the desk. Directly in front of the judge were two desks, one for each side of the lawsuit. They were about twenty feet away from the judge and five feet apart from each other. The attorneys were separated from the "audience" by a wooden railing. As soon as each prospective juror entered the courtroom, both groups of attorneys began furiously taking notes on every detail of the jurors' mannerisms, facial expressions, body language, and general demeanor. With every case, it is particularly important to pay the closest possible attention to the reactions of potential jurors when the judge reads aloud the summary of the case. During the jury selection phase of my trial, I remember there was an older woman, who immediately started to shake her head, roll her eyes and whisper to the woman sitting beside her as soon as the judge read the gist of the trial. When my attorneys saw her reaction, they concluded that she would be unsympathetic to my plight and, therefore, they did not want her on the jury.

The process of selecting a jury can take several hours. First, the judge reads out a list of questions, the answer to any one of which could potentially exclude someone from serving on the jury, questions such as "do you know the plaintiff or anyone associated with the plaintiff?" "Do you know the defendant or anyone associated with the defendant?" "Have you or anyone you know ever been a victim of medical malpractice?" "Are you or anyone you know involved in the medical profession?" Some who raise their hands to these questions are immediately excused. Others are called before the judge for additional questioning. And so the process continues until, eventually, you have twelve people sitting to the left of the judge. These twelve people will sit in judgment over the case you present and determine the merits of your case.

After the jury selection, the trial begins. So it was with my trial. First came the opening statements from each of the attorneys. On my side was Gary Freeman as lead counsel. Marian Riedy acted as his co-counsel. Gary was a slightly built man, standing about five feet eight inches tall. He had a smallish round face, with penetrating eyes that could look right through you and pierce the depths of a witness's soul. His co-counsel, Marian Riedy, was also of slight build, about five feet six inches tall. The thin, gaunt features of her face were contrasted with her larger-than-life and extraordinarily vivacious personality. You couldn't help but cheer her on and smile as she made mincemeat out of some of the witnesses on the hospital's side or summarily dismissed their testimony with a wave of her hand.

Representing GWUMC was Brian Nash. In stark contrast to Gary Freeman, Mr. Nash appeared as a large, jovial Santa Claus-type figure. Looking at him, it was difficult for me to imagine that this appealing man represented my adversary. The co-counsel for GWUMC was a man named Stuart Herschfeld, of whose appearance I have no clear recollection. Understandably, what Mr. Herschfeld looked like wasn't my concern. Brian Nash and the ammunition that he might have in his arsenal to destroy my case was what I worried about.

Gary Freeman began,[2] "Ladies and Gentlemen of the jury. On May 7, 1990, Cynthia Paddock entered the hospital to undergo what is considered by most medical experts to be a fairly routine brain operation to correct a condition known as hydrocephalus, commonly referred to as water on the brain. Ostensibly, the surgery was without incident. In reality, however, a blood clot formed on Ms. Paddock's brain, which developed and expanded over the course of four and one-half hours following the surgery. We have prepared a video to help you visualize what happened. In this video, you will see that as the bleed progresses, it strips the inner lining of the skull, known as the dura, away from the skull wall. The bleed then begins to compress the brain, shifting the brain to the left as it enlarges. The brain begins to buckle. In the final stage of this compression, the cortex or center of the brain begins

---

[2] Gary's opening statement included a preview of a great deal of medical information and technicalities regarding the liability of an employer for an employee, and other matters that were essential to my case, but do not stand out in my memory and so are not recorded here.

to cut off oxygen to the brain, sending the patient into cardiac arrest.

"The evidence will show that all these events have signs and symptoms associated with them. For example, as the patient's pain levels increase dramatically the patient starts asking for increased amounts of codeine to counteract this. The record will show that this is exactly what happened to Ms. Paddock. The record will likewise show that when Ms Paddock's brain nearly collapsed in on itself and she went into respiratory failure, she sustained serious and permanent neurological injuries as a result."

Gary continued. "It was in the Neurological Concentrated Care Unit (NCCU) that the hemorrhage became massive and clinical signs and symptoms of the enlarging clot developed. We will prove that these signs and symptoms went undetected because the nurse in charge of the NCCU, Barbara Boston, was negligent and failed to notice the signs of increased intracranial pressure (ICP). By the time she did notice the signs and notified the resident on call, the bleed had filled about one-quarter of the total volume of the skull, equivalent to eighteen ounces of blood.

"Through the testimony of experts in neurology and critical care nursing, we will prove that there must have been clinical signs and symptoms of Ms. Paddock's expanding blood clot, such as a change in alertness, headache, asymmetry of motor function and papillary changes, which were evident while she was in the NCCU and which a George Washington University Medical Center employee, nurse Barbara Boston, should have, but failed, to recognize. Minutes counted. It was the failure on the part of nurse Boston to identify these signs and symptoms and appropriately respond to the crisis that caused Ms. Paddock's permanent brain damage. The evidence will show that the defendant's employee provided substandard care and was negligent, and that Ms. Paddock's injuries were caused by that same negligence. We will also prove that Ms. Paddock was seriously and permanently damaged as a direct result of the defendant's negligence, and ask that you award her monetary damages to compensate for her injuries.

"Specifically, plaintiff's side will prove that the defendant violated standards of care and caused permanent neurological injury to Ms. Paddock as follows:

"Hospital personnel failed to timely and appropriately recognize and treat clinical signs and symptoms of an enlarging epidural hemorrhage from about 12:00 noon when plaintiff was transferred to the NCCU on May 7, 1990, and up to the time the neurosurgical resident arrived and began life-saving procedures at approximately 2:35 P.M.

"The Hospital failed to adequately train Nurse Barbara Boston to insure she had the nursing competency to work alone in the NCCU, to recognize signs and symptoms of increasing intracranial pressure (ICP) and appropriately respond to an enlarging epidural hemorrhage.

"The facts pertinent to this case are as follows:

"Ms. Paddock underwent the prescribed shunt procedure at The George Washington University Medical Center on May 7, 1990. She was sent to the Post-Anesthesia Care Unit (PACU) aka recovery room at 9:40 A.M. At 9:55 A.M., she was noted to be awake and oriented. At 10:35 A.M., she received codeine for pain and was noted to be nauseated. At 11:00 A.M. and again at 11:30 A.M., she was noted to be alert and oriented. At noon, Ms. Paddock was transferred to the NCCU. Shortly after her arrival, she was visited briefly by her parents and Dr. Laws. Her mother commented that she seemed 'awfully sleepy.' At 12:20 P.M., she received medication for pain and nausea. At 1:00 P.M., Nurse Boston indicated that she had conducted a neurological examination by checking boxes on the nursing flow chart. The nursing progress note indicates only 'no change in patient at this time.' Question? Did the nurse in charge of her care actually perform the required neurological examination?

"Barbara Boston was assigned to care for Ms. Paddock and one other patient in the four-patient unit. She testified that she went to lunch between 1:00 P.M. and 2:00 P.M. She is unable to identify the nurse who relieved her. Nurse Boston testified in her deposition that when she returned from lunch, she stood at the foot of Ms. Paddock's bed and 'saw that she was breathing regularly as if in a sleep state.' Rather than conduct the required hourly neurological assessment on Ms. Paddock, she went to the other patient's bed and spent twenty minutes at his bed performing a check of that patient's glucose level before returning to Ms. Paddock.

"At 2:20 P.M., Nurse Boston finally got around to conducting a neurological assessment of Ms. Paddock. She observed her to be stuporous, with her left arm at a twenty degree angle to her body, with her elbow turned tightly into her chest, commonly referred to as posturing. Her left pupil was also dilated. This change in level of consciousness, with posturing and unilateral papillary changes, are classic signs of brain stem compression.

When Nurse Boston could not awaken Ms. Paddock, she called the neurosurgical resident, who arrived 'within minutes.' She took no steps to render aid to Ms. Paddock until the resident arrived. She just stood there, looking at the patient. In his deposition, the resident testified that he was called because Nurse Boston could not awaken Ms. Paddock. He arrived within 'a minute or so' and observed the patient to be in respiratory failure, with her left pupil nonreactive. He immediately called a Code, administered life-saving drugs and placed a tube down her throat so she could breath. Ms Paddock was rushed down to x-ray for a CT scan, which showed a massive epidural hemorrhage. Thereafter, she was taken to the operating room for an emergency craniotomy to remove the blood clot. Saline solution was injected into her brain cavity to gradually recompress her brain and restore it to its normal size and shape.

"Ms. Paddock remained in The George Washington University Medical Center for approximately three months. Her hospital course was complicated by several other brain surgeries, a brain infection known as meningitis, seizures, and insertion of a stomach tube for feedings, because she couldn't swallow without choking herself. As a direct result of the brain stem compression and the subsequent operations, she sustained paralysis on her left side and suffers from severe cognitive and behavioral deficits."

Then came the opening statement from the defense:

Brian Nash's opening statement was a repudiation of the claims made by my attorney. This was not surprising. He began, "This case comes down to three principal issues: (1)What occurred during a two hour and twenty minute interval between 12:00 P.M. and 2:20 P.M. on May 7, 1990 and (2) should anything have been done to intervene earlier and stop the hemorrhage, and (3) if intervention had come earlier, would it have made any difference?" A follow up to that question was at what point should the bleed have been detected and why wasn't it detected?

Mr. Nash continued his opening statement, listing the major points of dispute between the two sides.

"At dispute is (1) whether any agent or employee of the hospital failed to timely and appropriately recognize and treat the clinical signs and symptoms of an enlarging epidural hemorrhage when plaintiff was transferred to the NCCU at about 12:00 noon on May 7, 1990, and up to the time (2:35 P.M.) the neurosurgical resident arrived and began life-saving procedures. (2) Was Nurse Boston adequately trained to work alone in the NCCU? (3) Were there any signs and symptoms of an enlarging epidural hemorrhage prior to the time Nurse Boston recognized that the plaintiff's neurological condition had changed at 2:20 P.M.? and (4) Was the most likely cause of plaintiff's brain infection the emergency shunt tap and/or emergency craniotomy on May 7, 1990, as contended by the plaintiff, or was the most likely cause of plaintiff's brain infection the initial surgery, the emergency craniotomy, or any of the other four operations that followed the initial one?"

And so the trial continued as most trials do, with witness testimony for my side saying one thing and the defense witnesses disputing our claims.

The second major event that stands out in my mind is when my mother took the stand. My attorney had strategically timed this appearance to come just before he planned to call me as a witness. My lawyer's reasoning behind this maneuver was that my mother and I look quite a bit alike. The jurors could project in their mind what I might look like some thirty years down the road. Secondly, it was late in the day. I was going to be tired. Consequently, my thought processes would be slower, my speech slower, and my movements shakier. In short, I might actually look and behave more like the brain-damaged person I was, my appearance to the contrary notwithstanding. Third, and most importantly, my mother can be a very emotional woman, especially when reliving the horrible events of May 7, 1990 when she almost lost her youngest child. If you are looking to garner the sympathy of the jury, she's the woman you want on the witness stand. The strategy worked.

As my mother approached the witness stand, she glanced at the jury with that warm, inviting smile that she wears so well.

Mr. Freeman began, "Mrs. Paddock, please describe for the jury what occurred the day of the surgery."

"Well, we got up about 4:30 A.M., got into a taxi and accompanied Cynthia to the hospital."

"What did you do and whom did you see upon arriving at the hospital?"

"I don't really remember seeing anyone in particular. We took Cynthia upstairs where someone came to get her prepped for surgery."

"And did you then return home?"

"No, we stayed in the hospital while the surgery was taking place, in the waiting area."

"And did you see Dr. Laws or any of the people who participated in the surgery that day?"

"We saw Dr. Laws when Cynthia was transferred into the NCCU. We had not seen him before that time. In fact, we waited and waited and waited for someone to contact us to let us know that the surgery was over, but no one ever did."

"Now, did this seem odd to you?"

"Well, yes, it definitely did. I remember when my husband had operations done in Tulsa, where we live. There was a special area where you could wait. The doctor called me and told me the surgery went all right and that my husband was in the recovery room. And then they told me that they would notify me when he was to be moved to his room. There was constant communication between the doctor and the patient's family. I know George Washington University Medical Center is a big hospital in a big city, but I expected a similar type of treatment."

Gary stopped at this point and turned to look at the jury as if to say, "And you wonder why people prefer small town hospitals."

He continued, addressing my mother in a tone of voice that was fraught with an air of disbelief. "And this similar type of treatment that you expected, did it ever occur?"

"No, it didn't. There were other doctors coming down to the waiting room and talking to *their* patients, but Dr. Laws never showed up."

"And so what happened after that?"

"Well, finally, knowing that she had been scheduled for surgery at 7:30 A.M. and it was nearly noon, I started to get concerned because we hadn't heard anything. So we started calling and calling, but no one would tell us anything. Finally, on our last call, they told us that she was being moved to the NCCU and we could go up and see her."

"And when you got up to the NCCU was Dr. Laws already there?"

"No."

"What happened after you got to the NCCU?"

"Well, we came in and I asked if Dr. Laws was there. I wanted to meet him because we had never met him."

"Did you speak to Cynthia at that time?"

"No. We went over to her bedside and I don't remember exactly what we did, but I remember thinking to myself that she was awfully sleepy for someone who had just been released from the recovery room."

"Objection, foundation," from Mr. Nash.

"Sustained," from Judge Zeldon.

"I will rephrase. Mrs. Paddock, what if any experience do you have with patients and their condition after release from the recovery room?"

"Well, I've had two surgeries, and as I said, my husband has had one, and I remember what condition I was in when I was sent to my room after recovery. I was a lot more lucid than she was."

"At what point did you speak with Dr. Laws?"

"I don't remember exactly. He just came in at some point, introduced himself, and told us that the surgery had gone well."

"And then what happened?"

"Well, at some point during this time, it was indicated to us that she would be moved later to her own room and considering her sleepiness and the fact that we had been up since 4:30 A.M. ourselves, we decided to head back to where we were staying, get some lunch and some rest, and then come back later, when she would be in her room and presumably more awake."

"At what point did you receive notification from the hospital that something had happened?"

"We never did. We found out when we came back to the hospital."

"And at what time was that, approximately?"

"About 5:30 P.M."

"Tell the jury in your own words what happened."

"Well, we came up on the elevator and when I got off the elevator I looked down the hall. As we were starting down the hall, there was this one nurse that I recognized and I saw her glance at us and then whisper something to somebody next to her. I don't remember exactly what it was, a gesture, a look on her face, I don't know. But it just hit me that something had gone wrong. Call it mother's intuition."

"Please continue," Gary said, gently, with full appreciation that my mother was about to relive one of the most horrible moments a mother could endure.

"Well we proceeded down the hall and started to enter Cynthia's room and they told us that she had to go back into surgery because she had started to bleed."

"And what were your thoughts at that moment?"

"Well, at first I thought they were talking about her bleeding around the abdomen, because the shunt drains into the abdomen. When they said, no, she was bleeding into her brain, my heart fell into my stomach. Know what I mean?" And at this my mother's eyes began to tear up and it looked to me like she was trembling.

"I do indeed. I'm sure we can all imagine how you felt."

"What happened next?"

"I can't remember exactly. I was in shock. They told us to go back to the waiting room, which we did, until Dr. Laws and Dr. VonDerSchmidt showed up."

"And what did Dr. Laws say to you when he arrived?"

"All I remember was Dr. Laws saying, 'We almost lost her.' And I remember thinking, 'how could this have happened? This was supposed to have been a routine operation.' A parent is not supposed to outlive their child. I was devastated."

"Thank you, Mrs. Paddock. I'm sorry to make you relive what was obviously a very painful and traumatic period in your life. Next, I'd like you to describe for the jury how Cynthia progressed over time. However, do you need a break first or can we continue?"

"No. It's okay. Go on."

Gary continued his questioning.

"Mrs. Paddock, please describe for the jury how Cynthia was when she finally awakened from her coma and what progress you saw in her different rehabilitation programs and what limitations she still has."

"Well, she was dismissed from Magee Rehabilitation Hospital (Magee) on October 18, 1990."

"Magee was the first rehabilitation program she was in, correct?"

"Correct. It is located in Philadelphia, Pennsylvania."

"What was her condition when she was dismissed from Magee?"

"Well, when she was dismissed from Magee in October, she was like a baby. I was her primary care giver. I had to toilet train her, because she was still in diapers and do a significant amount of physical therapy with her. Magee had given us some materials for speech, occupational and cognitive therapy, but I mainly focused on the physical aspects of her injury. I was determined that she was going to have full use of her left arm again, especially because that was her writing arm."

"What was wrong with her arm?"

"Cynthia's arm was bent at a twenty degree angle from her body with her elbow turned tightly into her chest and completely useless. It had been in that position for so long that the muscles had atrophied and the tendons had shortened. I focused on the exercises Magee had given us to try to straighten her arm back out. It was tremendously painful for her. She would cry and beg me to stop, but I just kept moving ahead. I was determined that my daughter was not going to stay a cripple."

"Anything else you particularly remember from that time?"

"She would also sleep a great deal, like babies do. She would take a nap for about two hours in the morning around 10:00 A.M. and then again in the afternoon around 2:00 P.M. or 3:00 P.M. And then go to bed around 9:00 P.M. As I said, she slept a lot!"

"How was she in terms of her physical abilities?"

"Physically, she was very weak. She had entered the hospital at roughly 130 pounds. She was ninety pounds by the time she left Magee. She could barely walk and then for only short distances."

"And how would you describe her emotional state of mind while at Magee or after leaving there?"

"I remember that emotionally she was like a child as well. She would get very teary and sometimes just bawl uncontrollably at the slightest thing. I think it was principally from frustration and her keen awareness that what she mentally and physically had been able to do prior to her injury, she could no longer do. I'm sure it was also embarrassing for her to be twenty-six years of age and in diapers. After she got out of diapers, I know she had a couple of accidents in her rehabilitation program in Dallas where she didn't make it to the bathroom in time and soiled herself. I know she was humiliated."

"Mrs. Paddock, just so the members of the jury can get an appreciation for what you mean when you say Cynthia was more emotional than usual, can you describe a specific incident you remember?"

"Yes, I can. It was the day we came back to Magee after having been away for two weeks."

"Why were you away for two weeks?"

"The staff at Magee asked us to go back to Tulsa for two weeks to get our affairs in order and to give them time to work one-on-one with Cynthia without the distraction of having her parents there."

"And so what happened on the day you returned?" Gary asked this question with all the certainty of knowing what the answer would be and you could tell by the gleam in his eye that he knew the emotional impact of my mother's next response would be deep.

"We were riding up in the elevator with her and she looked at us, with that blank, dawn-of-the-dead stare she had acquired since the injury."

"Dawn-of-the-dead stare?"

"Yes. You know that look where two black pupils are staring out at you straight ahead with no emotion and with no obvious signs of any brain activity going on behind them? You've seen the movie?"

"Okay. I understand. Go on."

"So she looked at us and calmly asked how long we were staying. We told her, 'until they tell us we can take you home.' She looked up at the heavens and cried out, 'Oh, thank you God.' And then just collapsed into a sobbing heap."

There wasn't a dry eye in the court room after my mother's testimony, including my own.

An integral part of my mother's testimony was the issue of timing. As the defense attorney for GWUMC said in his opening statement, "This case comes down to what occurred during a two hour and twenty minute interval between 12:00 P.M. and 2:20 P.M. on May 7, 1990, whether anything could have been done to intervene earlier and stop the hemorrhage, and if intervention had come earlier, would it have made any difference?" A follow up to that question was at what point should the bleed have been detected and why wasn't it detected? The "when" was important. If the bleed had been discovered around 1:00 P.M., when the nurse supposedly checked in on me before going to lunch, as opposed to one hour and twenty minutes later after she had returned from lunch and finished up with the other patient, I would not have been left permanently brain damaged and paralyzed on the left side of my body. The nursing records indicated that "family" was visiting me at 12:00 noon, but my mother had testified in her deposition that she and my father had seen me between 1:30 P.M. and 2:00 P.M. and had met Dr. Laws at that time. So, if in fact Dr. Laws had been in there at 1:30 P.M. and didn't pick up any signs of the bleed, then I obviously could not have been in a critical stage at that time. And if I wasn't in a critical stage at that time, the nurse could not be held responsible for not picking up signs of increased intracranial pressure at 1:00 P.M., especially if the neurosurgeon himself hadn't noticed those signs.

My mother's testimony in her deposition was "confirmed" by my deposition testimony. In fact I was just repeating what I had learned of my condition from my mother. I really had no idea. I include an excerpt from that deposition:

Defense attorney, Brian Nash: "Has your mother told you anything about the day she saw you after the surgery in terms of the time of day?"

"I think it was around 1:30 P.M. or 2:00 P.M., because they had tickets to see the White House, thanks to our Congressman, and they had to pick the tickets up by 5:00 P.M. So, they decided to go home and take a nap first, then go to the Congressman's office and then return to the hospital. I think they told me it was around 12:30 P.M. Or maybe it was around 1:30 P.M. or 2:00 P.M. when they returned. I'm not really sure." (In retrospect, it was fortunate that my deposition testimony was so undependable. There could have been nothing more helpful to my case than the unreliable testimony of the brain-injured plaintiff to play havoc with the issue of timing. In the end, that kind of testimony probably bolstered my case more than hurt it, because it was clear I didn't have any idea of the time and so the only thing left to salvage was my mother's deposition testimony.)

The way my attorney rehabilitated my mother's deposition testimony was brilliant, to say the least. The entire time he had her on the witness stand, asking her questions about my condition, about how dependent I was on both my parents, he never once asked what time she and my father had come up to the NCCU to see me. He left that for the co-counsel for the defense, who he knew would bring up the topic and the opposing attorney indeed stepped right into the trap.

True to expectations, on cross examination, the co-counsel for GWUMC, Stuart Herschfeld, began to quiz my mother regarding her recollection of the time she and my father first saw me.

Mr. Herschfeld began, "Mrs. Paddock, when you went up to the NCCU, do you have a sense of what time that was approximately?"

"Well, as I said in my deposition, I think it was sometime after 1:30 P.M. But I really don't remember exactly."

"What helps you place it at least after 1:30 P.M.?"

"Because that was approximately when I called the last time and was told that we could go up to see her."

"Do you have any sense of how long you were in there with her?"

"No, I don't, but it couldn't have been very long. She was groggy and unresponsive, so we decided to return home and give her a chance to wake up."

Nothing there. "No further questions." Having relinquished his witness, he had no further recourse for follow up questioning.

And then it was Gary's turn to redirect.

"Mrs. Paddock, you stated in your deposition that you arrived at the NCCU about 1:30 P.M."

"That is what I said."

"Well let's examine that," Gary said, with a barely perceptible smile. He then completely backed into the time frame, equipped with a flow chart of everything my mother claimed she and my father had done from the time they first saw me to the time when they returned to the hospital "at about 5:30 P.M." On the flow chart was a column indicating the amount of time required for each activity. It was clear from this time line that there was no way my parents could have accomplished everything they claimed they had done in only four hours.

"Given this time line, Mrs. Paddock, do you see any possible way you could have accomplished all this in just four hours?"

"Well, no I don't."

"So, given what we have just gone through. Do you still maintain that you saw Cynthia in the NCCU and spoke with Dr. Laws around 1:30 P.M.?"

"No, I was obviously wrong. It would have to have been earlier."

Brilliant! Slam dunk! Home run! The ball is out of the park! As a spectator sitting on the sidelines, it was truly an amazing legal maneuver to witness.

The third memorable event in the trial for me was the testimony of two neuropsychologists and the expert report filed on behalf of Estelle Davis, a vocational-rehabilitation counselor. The first neuropsychologist to appear for the plaintiff was Terry Shaw. Dr. Shaw had been born and raised near McAlester, Oklahoma and was known to be a bit eccentric. Sporting black cowboy boots, a bojangle tie and long, curly black locks, his dress and appearance were in keeping with his reputation. He certainly didn't fit somebody's image of a neuropsychologist. Gary began his direct examination with a few preliminary questions to qualify Dr. Shaw as an expert witness.

"Dr. Shaw, could you please describe your educational and professional background?"

"Sure. I attended undergraduate school at Oklahoma State University from 1966 to 1972. Graduated with a bachelor's degree in psychology. Accepted a National Institutes of Mental Health (NIMH) federal trainingship fellowship at the University of Houston, which I attended from 1972 to 1975. I earned my master's degree, and in 1976, I finished my doctoral degree."

"Where are you licensed to practice and in what hospitals do you have privileges?"

"I hold licenses in the states of Texas and Oklahoma, and have hospital privileges in a variety of hospitals in the area that allow me to see patients and I have a few consulting gigs in the area."

"Any articles, essays or other publications that are pertinent to the opinions you will be expressing today?"

"I have an extensive list of publications that I have been involved in. The two most pertinent ones for today's testimony would be the two articles I wrote on neuro imaging studies in different types of neuropathology, including stroke and head injury."

"Thank you, Dr. Shaw."

"Your honor. I proffer this witness as an expert in the field of neuropsychology and qualified to express opinions in the area of his expertise."

The judge inquired, "Any objection?"

The judge continued, "Hearing no objection on the record, the jury is instructed that Dr. Shaw has been qualified to testify as an expert witness. At the close of the case, I will give you instructions on how you are to consider any opinions expressed by an expert witness in reaching your verdict."

With those preliminaries over, Gary began his line of questioning.

"Dr. Shaw, it is my understanding that you treated Ms. Paddock during her time at the Kaiser Rehabilitation Center in Tulsa, Oklahoma from March to June 1992. Correct?"

"That is correct. I administered one battery of neuropsychological tests on Ms. Paddock."

"What are these tests designed to evaluate?"

"These tests are used to determine the nature and extent of a person's neurological deficits and how these deficits may have an impact on a person's social and professional future."

Gary continued. "Could you briefly describe your test findings?"

"Well, in fact I did two exams on Ms. Paddock, within a year and a half of each other and I must say there was a substantial change in her neurological condition between the two exams."

"Do you have any explanation for the change?"

"I believe I do. The first test was given to her in April 1992, just before she returned to Washington, D. C. to resume her studies. The second exam was given to her in December 1993, approximately four months after she had had another surgical operation. I think the surgery, which constituted another assault on her brain so to speak, had a lot to do with the deterioration of her neurological deficits."

"Would you please explain the nature of Miss Paddock's deficits, the continuing problems she is dealing with, and what impact you believe that her requiring yet another brain operation has had on her?"

"Sure." Dr. Shaw then began his commentary. "Given her achievement levels and some of her word skills and word knowledge, it can be assumed that Ms. Paddock's IQ pre-injury was in the above-average to superior range. Six months post-injury, testing shows that Ms. Paddock had the IQ of a vegetable. Although she has made significant progress, she still has numerous deficits she is forced to contend with, and which have had a significant impact on her ability to excel both personally and professionally. At present, her verbal IQ is still very much in the superior range, while her performance IQ is in the average range. Specifically, her executive skills – the ability to sequence back and forth between cognitive tasks, to shift back and forth, to keep track of multiple channels of information at the same time, and the ability to be fairly flexible cognitively - have been severely compromised."

In comparing the results of the tests that were a year and a half apart, Dr. Shaw testified that he saw a marked decrease in my cognitive abilities. He elaborated, "Ms. Paddock is not efficient in many aspects of her information processing skills. Her attention skills were a little less efficient than they were in 1992. What continues to be striking is that those deficits which were most dramatic in the earlier testing in 1992, have actually gotten worse instead of improved. This is most likely the result of the recent shunt procedure in 1993."

"What is your prognosis for her continued recovery?"

"After two years, there is virtually no hope that her left extremity is ever going to move with any agility ever again. I believe she has achieved most of the biological and physical recovery that she is going to achieve." He continued, "Since she was first tested by me in 1992, Cynthia has shown some decreases in terms of her ability to process nonverbal pitch rhythm perceptual qualities. Her visual attention skills and visual search skills have decreased dramatically. Again, I have noted some worsening of the original deficits. Her visual memory has gotten worse and her math skills have gotten significantly worse. When I saw her in 1992, she was in the 97th percentile on the rope math tests. Those scores have dropped to the 53rd percentile. Her dexterity in her left extremity has also gotten significantly worse."

"Is it your opinion, Doctor, that her deficits will continue to erode?"

"It is my opinion that Cynthia will always be at risk of losing skills in the areas that have been already damaged by the brain injury. In the face of any additional intervening problems, it is tough to say where she'll end up. Her deficits will only become more dramatic as she ages."

"What is your prognosis for Ms. Paddock?"

"Cynthia clearly has superior language ability. She clearly has sublevel nonverbal processing skills. The typical scenario for individuals like her is that they can succeed fairly well in a structured environment, such as academia, where the teacher tells you when and in what sequence and what to do and what to accomplish. Where these individuals with these types of deficits struggle is in the unstructured settings, where they have to deal with time and space continually, being able to arrange their schedule, to accomplish things with efficiency. They are basically pretty poor time managers. They lack the ability to structure their daily routine in an efficient manner. So, it takes them longer to do things.

"That has to do with the fact that time is a nonverbal entity and their ability to structure first step, second step, last step internally is also a nonverbal entity. What happens frequently is that individuals like Cynthia do fine when they are in school, but once they get out of school they fall flat on their face, because there is nobody to provide the structure.

"It remains to be seen if this happens in Cynthia's case. However, this leads me into what I see as a more significant concern, and that is with Cynthia's ability to operate successfully on a social level."

"What do you mean by that?"

"Social interchange, social interaction, is largely nonverbal. It's nonverbal from the standpoint of facial expressions, body gestures, and body language. Even the point of inflection and intonation in voices is important. The age old problem of 'it's not what you say, but how you say it.' Cynthia shows problems with pitch perception, which generally leads into problems with prosody, otherwise known as the issue of 'it's not what you say, but how you say it'.

"Cynthia also shows some problems with affect recognition, which means she will have problems reading nonverbal cues. In fact, she has stated on numerous occasions that she has problems understanding how people are feeling and she has to point blank ask them how they are feeling. Are you mad at me? Is everything all right? Questions of that nature.

"These problems of structure and problems associated with nonverbal problem-solving, particularly as it relates to social interchange, can create a pretty significant deficit in terms of marketability if in fact your job or your intended profession is to meet the public." He continued, "I anticipate that she will continue to be inefficient in a nonverbal sense and that, as it impacts her socially, her failure in the social realm, her inability to navigate a social relationship with somebody of the opposite sex in particular, will cause her to withdraw just as her inability to navigate in an occupational role that is dependent on the skills she no longer has will cause her to withdraw."

"Do you think she is suicidal?"

"Yes. I think Cynthia is having a very difficult time accepting and adapting to her deficits. She was a high achiever. And she's not only unable to achieve at that same high level anymore, but she's not able to achieve in a social context either. She will need a lot of emotional and psychological support, probably for the rest of her life."

"Thank you, Dr. Shaw."

"Thank you."

And then came the testimony of Dr. Arthur Mac-Neil Horton, the psychotherapist I had been seeing since August 1993 and up to the time of the trial in April 1995. I had been referred to Dr. Horton by Dr. Shaw after a break up that had left me emotionally devastated. In contrast to Terry Shaw, Dr. Horton did fit the image of a neuropsychologist. He arrived in the courtroom wearing a dark blue suit and his manner was very staid and serious. He was called to further bolster Terry Shaw's findings.

As with previous expert witnesses, the jury was first presented with a summary of Dr. Horton's credentials in order to qualify him as an expert.

Gary Freeman began, "Dr. Horton, briefly describe for the jury your educational and professional background, please."

"Well, I have been a practicing neuropsychologist for almost 18 years. I received my B.A. from the University of Virginia in 1969 and my M.A. from the same institution in 1971. I then did an internship at the Veterans Administration Medical Centers in Richmond and Charleston, South Carolina where I worked in a neurology ward and learned how to administer the standard Halstead-Reitan Neuropsychological Test Battery. I also performed a rather innovative study on using behavioral modification with a neurologically-impaired patient."

"This test battery you just mentioned. Is this the same battery of tests that Dr. Shaw twice performed on Miss Paddock?"

"That is correct."

"Please continue."

"In addition to those stints, I also worked in outpatient psychiatry and spent some time in a drug treatment unit and some time treating patients with spinal cord injuries. The majority of my time, however, was in an outpatient neurology unit under the aegis of the Medical College of Virginia."

"From 1977 on, where did you work?"

"I worked at a variety of places. I worked at The Citadel, a private military school for boys, for one year. Then I took a position at the Veterans Administration hospital in Martinsburg, West Virginia for just under five years and then was offered a position at the Baltimore Veterans Administration hospital where I stayed for eight years. Finally, I was offered a position at the National Institutes of Health's Institute on Drug Abuse in 1990. That is where I am currently."

"Your resume indicated that you are licensed in the District of Columbia, Maryland, South Carolina, Virginia and West Virginia. Are these licenses still valid today?"

"Yes."

"Thank you, Dr. Horton. Your honor, I proffer Dr. Horton as an expert in neuropsychology and qualified to express opinions in the area of his expertise."

"Any objection?" the judge asked the members of the opposing counsel.

Hearing no objection, Dr. Arthur MacNeil Horton was sworn in as an expert witness. And then Gary proceeded with the bulk of the questioning.

In a very matter-of-fact tone of voice, Gary addressed Dr. Horton.

"Dr. Horton, could you tell the jury in your own words how you would classify Cynthia in terms of her intelligence, her cognitive deficits and her future personal and professional prospects?"

"My pleasure."

Leaning forward, his back to the judge so that he could squarely face the jury and with his face taking on the appearance of a teacher patiently explaining a complicated mathematical concept, Dr. Horton began his testimony. "Cynthia had above average to superior intelligence pre-injury. As a result of her injury, she has marked and considerable diminution in IQ. Verbal IQ is controlled by the left hemisphere. She is impaired much more in the right hemisphere. Her difficulties with visual, spatial, problem-solving, and organizing skills are permanent. Two years is the normal window for these things to improve. Work that requires use of both hemispheres will be difficult for her, because she can't put them together.

"Cynthia has visual spatial difficulty in processing objects. For example, a cat went by and she remarked what a cute dog. In other words, she misperceived a cat as a dog. In terms of cognitive deficits, she has a lot of trouble with space and time, difficulties with problem-solving, and visual and spatial deficits, which affect her ability to perceive and process information. She has trouble reading people's faces and interpreting what people are telling her. She will often have to point blank ask them what are you thinking, what are you feeling, are you mad at me? These types of deficits will obviously translate into emotional and social problems and difficulty making friends and maintaining relationships.

"Unfortunately for Cynthia, her left hemisphere was not as impaired and so her language skills are still intact. I say, "unfortunately," because the fact that her language skills are still intact can be deceptive and lead to a false sense of security. The trouble starts when she takes a job, which on paper she is qualified for, but which in reality is beyond her capabilities.

The Courtroom Drama

"The future I see for her is one in which she is dealing with a minimal set of activities within prescribed and
set routines. She will continue to suffer from environ-
mental stress due to her inability to make her abilities
meet demands. This will inevitably make her depressed
and anxious, more likely to make bad judgments and
more likely to be pessimistic. The best that can be hoped
for is a situation in which she is able to maintain some
sort of balance. She doesn't handle surprises well or the
occasional interruption in her routine."

Additional commentary on the future that lay before
me came through the expert report of Estelle Davis, a
vocational-rehabilitation counselor. I had originally met
with Estelle in April 1994 for an evaluation in my attorney's office. The report she wrote on our meeting and her
assessment of my career potential was like a checklist of
the hopes and dreams that were destroyed by this tragedy
and presented a somber and depressing picture of my
future. This expert report was read aloud to the jury and
submitted into evidence.

Ms. Davis wrote: "Cynthia is now almost four years
post insult. Although she has made significant progress in
her rehabilitation, she continues to have multiple deficits
that, according to medical doctors and neuropsychologists, are permanent. These include:

- Left–side paralysis resulting in sensory and
  motor deficits and requiring the use of a
  brace on the left lower extremity, and the use
  of a cane for balance.
- Diminution in cognitive function resulting in
  (a) short term memory problems, (b) nonverbal problem solving difficulties, (c) im-

37

pairment in extracting social meaning from non-verbal cues, (d) problems with tone discrimination, (e) inefficient visual memory, (f) problems with scheduling, time management and accomplishing things with efficiency, (g) inability to grasp the whole picture
- Loss of self confidence
- Psychological depression with suicidal potential
- Continued need for anti-epileptic medication

"Prior to her insult in May, 1990, judging from her accomplishments, Ms. Paddock was a very high functioning individual. Academically, she completed her undergraduate work at Amherst College, which according to Baron's Profile of American Colleges, ranks among the 'most competitive.' She has also studied at other prestigious schools, including the London School of Economics and The Johns Hopkins University School of Advanced International Studies.

"From her past experience in school, foreign travel and her work settings, I must assume that prior to her insult, Ms. Paddock was an independent, outgoing individual who was not only bright, but was socially astute and able to apply her knowledge effectively. The deposition transcript of James Montgomery, a former employer and Foreign Service officer, which was given to me, supports this. He stated that 'she was an entirely plausible Foreign Service Officer – that she had the intellect, the poise, and the memory to end up high on the roster.'

"Ms. Paddock has an educational and work background that prepares her to work and interact with other high-functioning people in the United States and abroad. She is fluent in Russian, and has studied other foreign languages. Her training has prepared her academically to work in jobs that require the ability to remember and synthesize all types of material, and to be able to think and respond rapidly 'on her feet'.

"It is my opinion that absent the stroke and related brain injury, Ms. Paddock would have had numerous career opportunities available to her. She would have finished her graduate work in May 1991 and within one year would have had an appointment with the Foreign Service or some other public and private agency dealing with economic interests abroad. She could likely have had an entry level salary of $29,000 per year in the public sector to $65,000 in the private sector.

"Cynthia's background is in a geographic area where competent people are in high demand. Given her background, her fluency in Russian and with a master's degree she could expect rapid advancement to high level salaries within five years. Pre-injury, Cynthia clearly had, at an early age, the potential to earn $95,000 - $110,000 per year. In addition, most private sector jobs offer a regular bonus of 15% to 20% per year, plus excellent benefits.

"As Cynthia is now, her cognitive deficits will be problematic for her not only in employment, but in everyday social function, and will keep her from using her skills at the level for which she has been trained.

"For example, her difficulty in tone discrimination will directly affect her facility and accuracy in learning new foreign languages. The impairment in her ability to recognize social cues and unspoken language, coupled with short-term memory problems pose a critical barrier to her chosen field in the Foreign Service and to positions of similar responsibility with other government agencies or private industry.

"In his deposition, Mr. Montgomery describes the need, as a Foreign Service Officer, to carry on conversations and figure out what's going on, and what is actually being said. He discusses the need to remember who you've made promises to, and the need to keep all of these things in your head. Ms. Paddock's brain injury has impaired the functions necessary to perform such activities.

"In addition to the cognitive deficits, Ms. Paddock has a significant physical deficit that manifests itself in a limp. This physical deficit limits her mobility, and will preclude any job requiring more than occasional walking or standing.

"Because of her limitations and deficits, it is my opinion that Ms. Paddock will not be able to work in the Foreign Service, or in any other job at the level for which she has been trained, either in this country or abroad.

"Cynthia has made a remarkable recovery from her original insult. She has retained good verbal skills and has been able to continue in school. She is employable, but at a much lower level than she would have been, absent the insult.

"With her intact verbal skills, she should be able to work in a structured setting where stress would be at a minimum. For example, most federal agencies, as well as state and local governments have publications departments, which would have positions that she could handle. Many jobs in procurement would also be appropriate.

With her education and background, her earnings would range between $22, 700 and $36,000 per year.

"It is also my opinion that if Ms. Paddock finds such employment, it is likely she will not be able to work to the usual retirement age, but will need to leave the work force five to ten years earlier, due to her physical problems.

"Let me conclude by stating that I have a major concern about her mental health, particularly at this point in her life. In my opinion, she is in a crisis period in her life, as she will finish school in May and must look for work. Considering her impairments, her job search could have several outcomes. She could find a job and not be able to perform at the level expected, or be frozen at entry level, unable to get promotions. She is also at risk for applying for positions and being continually turned down. In either of these scenarios, her depression could worsen and she may never be able to find work.

"Cynthia needs professional help with her job search. Considering the stressors in her life, it is imperative that Cynthia have vocational counseling that is separate and apart from the career guidance and placement offered by her school. Cynthia needs help from someone who understands the work world and her limitations and abilities, particularly with regard to the brain injury."

The testimony of Dr. Horton, Dr. Davis and Dr. Shaw was a veritable checklist of all that I had lost. Hearing it, I felt even more depressed and suicidal. I can imagine that some of you reading this can identify with the kind of despair and hopelessness in your own life that I felt at that point. "What was all my education for?" I asked myself. "What was all this hard work during rehabilitation for? To end up like this, with no hope and no future?" Well keep on reading. We will find that open door.

The fourth memorable event of my trial was the day Nurse Barbara Boston appeared in court. Nurse Boston was the nurse in charge of my care in the NCCU on May 7, 1990 and from all we could discover, the responsibility for what happened could be placed squarely at her feet. Her obviously inadequate education and training aside, her court room demeanor did not help the defense's case either. She certainly did not make an impression as a well-trained and experienced nurse.

Nurse Boston appeared as the first witness for the defense.

Assuming his characteristic affable smile and de- meanor, Brian Nash began the questioning of his first witness, "Miss Boston, briefly summarize for the jury your educational background."

"I attended Pensacola Junior College. There I ob- tained a general degree in business. I went back to Pensa- cola for nursing and went through approximately one year of nursing there. I changed schools to Jefferson Davis State Junior College in Brewton, Alabama where I completed my nursing degree. I have an R.N. associate degree as well."

"Is Jefferson Davis a two-year or four-year college?"

"Two year."

"How long did you attend Jefferson Davis to get your degree?"

"The actual time I was in classes was one year and six months."

"But in essence, you did receive a two-year associate's degree?"

"Yes."

"Why did you leave Pensacola Junior College and transfer to Jefferson Davis State College?"

"I didn't feel like I was learning the demanded material in the right time frame, because it was a very short summer term, so I wanted to return to Pensacola during the fall term and have more time to study the material. After I dropped out of the class, they told me I could not get back in because the fall term had already been filled. So, I changed schools."

"Why didn't you take a four-year R.N. program?"

"Because I had already spent time getting an associate degree. My parents were paying for my school and I didn't want to financially tax them."

I remember thinking to myself as I heard her testimony, "Oh, my God! This woman only had an associate's degree? She was clearly not qualified to be the sole person working in the NCCU. And to think GWUMC put this woman in charge of my care. It boggles the mind. Makes you think twice before putting your life into the hands of any hospital, doesn't it?"

The details of her background got worse. Brian Nash continued. "Miss Boston, have you had any college training other than your associate's degree during the past seven years from 1988 to March 1995?"

"I have attended a few classes at the University of West Florida and Pensacola to get some of the prerequisites for my B.S. out of the way."

"Are you actively pursuing a bachelor's degree in nursing at this point?"

"No, I'm not in any classes."

"When was the last time you took courses towards a bachelor's degree in nursing?"

"Maybe a year and a half, two years ago."

"Okay, let's move on."

The nightmare testimony continued. We were ultimately to learn that her only experience was working on the general surgical floor of a hospital in Pensacola, Florida. She was on the night staff in charge of generalized post-surgical patient care, "primarily abdominal surgeries and that sort of thing." She had had no specialized in-service training at any of the hospitals at which she had worked. When she arrived at GWUMC, her entire training consisted of being taught how to assess cranial nerves, receiving a videotape on EKG monitoring and being given a notebook covering a wide variety of topics. She had never worked on the neurosurgery floor before she arrived at GWUMC in 1989. The hospital placed her on the neurosurgery floor for two to three months and then assigned her to the NCCU. Her training for that specialized unit consisted of reading additional in-depth pamphlets on neurosurgery, receiving instruction on how to do a neurological assessment, attending a class on EKG for a week, following a more experienced nurse for a week or two until she learned the ropes and then she was left on her own.

Again, I thought, "Oh, my God."

The defense examination of Nurse Boston continued. Many of her responses ran the gamut from "I'm not sure" to "I don't remember". It was clear that she didn't remember many details of what she had studied, or what she had learned, or even the time frames when much of this occurred. Or at least that is what she testified to.

Brian Nash continued with his examination.

"Nurse Boston. I would like to turn your attention to the sequence of events of May 7, 1990."

"Do you remember being assigned to care for Ms. Paddock on that day?"

"Yes."

"What shift were you working that day?"

"According to the nursing notes that I received, I was either working a 7:00 A.M. to 3:00 P.M. shift or a 7:00 A.M. to 7:00 P.M. shift. I don't recall which."

"Do you have any recollection of how many patients there were in the NCCU during that shift?"

"Out of a total possible of four patients, there were two that day."

"How is it that you remember that?"

"I remember the events of that day."

"Okay. Nurse Boston, I'd like to turn your attention to what occurred during the specific time period of 12:00 noon to 2:20 P.M."

"What was the first thing you did after Miss Paddock arrived into the NCCU?"

"I don't remember exactly, but I would have taken vital signs on her and done a neuroassessment."

"Can you show the jury for me what all is involved in doing a neuroassessment?"

"Sure." Nurse Boston then stepped out of the witness box and standing before the jury, but facing Brian Nash, she conducted a simulated neuroassessment. From the looks on some of the juror's faces, Nurse Boston's so-called neuroassessment was so staged, it was not even believable. It made me sick just watching it.

"Thank you," said Mr. Nash enthusiastically and with a barely perceptible sigh of relief. "Please return to the witness stand.

"Nurse Boston, in your nursing note of 12 noon, you indicated that you had medicated the patient with Tigan, 200 milligrams."

"That is correct."

"What is Tigan used for?"

"Nausea."

"Did you administer any other medications?"

"She was complaining of pain, so I also gave her thirty milligrams of codeine."

Brian Nash continued.

"Nurse Boston, please tell me for the jury, did you take any vital signs for Miss Paddock and, if so, what were they?"

"According to my nursing notes, upon arriving in the NCCU at 12 noon, her blood pressure (BP) was 140/84. Her heart rate was 88. She had normal sinus rhythms. Her color was fair. Her respiratory rate was even and unlabored. She was voiding without difficulty."

"Did you observe anything that would cause you any alarm?"

"No. Nothing that would cause any alarm."

"Okay. Let's move on. At 1:00 P.M., did you conduct another neuroassessment on the patient?"

"Yes, I did."

"What did the neuroassessment show?"

"There was no change in patient status."

"What if anything in the medical record shows the results of your 1:00 P.M. neuroassessment?"

"There are check marks beside the 1:00 P.M. time slot, which means that there was no change in the patient's neurological status since the previous exam."

"Did you ever leave the patient unattended?"

"No."

"So you are absolutely sure there was no change in her status as of 1:00 P.M.?"

"That is correct."

"Do you have any doubt that you performed a neuroassessment at 1:00 P.M?"

"No I don't."

"Okay. Now I'd like to turn your attention to the nursing note you have at 12 noon where it indicates there was family visiting. Is there any chance that Dr. Laws could have been in during that time?"

"No. I would remember if he had been in."

"What about while you were at lunch? Any chance he may have come in during that time?"

"I seriously doubt it. If he had been in, the relief nurse would have told me."

"And as far as you can remember, no one mentioned this fact to you?"

"That is correct."

"When is the first time you ever observed any significant changes in Ms. Paddock's neurological status?"

"At 2:20 P.M., when I next checked her."

"Do you have any doubt as we sit here today, that you failed in any way to monitor Ms. Paddock as you had been taught and trained?"

"I have no doubt."

"Thank you, Nurse Boston. Your witness."

Then came the cross-examination of Nurse Boston by my attorney, Gary Freeman. Gary rose slowly from the table where he was seated and walked slowly and deliberately towards Nurse Boston. He looked at the jury as he approached the witness and then, in a level, measured and calculated tone of voice, he began his cross examination.

"Nurse Boston, we just heard you say that you have no doubt about some of the events of that day. That, in fact, you remember clearly the events of that day. Am I correct?"

"Correct."

"Nurse Boston, let's go over what you *don't* remember. You don't remember any details of the NCCU test nor the details of the test you had to take on the EKG, except you remember you had to take it twice, correct?"

"That's correct."

"You don't recall when you started in the NCCU, am I correct?"

"That's correct."

"You don't recall the name of the nurse that filled in for you when you went to lunch, correct?"

"Correct."

"You don't recall the number of nurses on the general neurosurgery floor nor the number of beds on the floor, correct?"

"That's correct."

"You have no recollection of your post-operative notes, correct?"

"Correct."

"You have no recollection of any protocols that existed for checking patients, correct?"

"Correct."

"You have no recollection today of the patient care plan that you had talked about in your deposition, is that correct?"

"Correct."

"You have no recollection of administering sixty milligrams of codeine; you say you only administered thirty milligrams, correct?"

"Correct."

"You have no recollection of Ms. Paddock's condition except that she was groggy, correct?"

"Correct."

"You have a note that family was visiting at 12:00 noon, but no recollection of who, exactly, was meant by family, correct?"

"Correct."

"You have no recollection of anyone telling you that Dr. Laws had come in to examine the patient, correct?"

"Correct."

"You have no recollection of the noon assessment you supposedly did. You have only hospital records to rely on for that, correct?"

"Correct."

"Regarding the 1:00 P.M. time frame in question, you do not recall whether you wrote a note at 1:00 P.M. rather than just using check marks, correct?"

"Correct."

"The only thing you remember when you returned from lunch at 2:00 P.M. is that Miss Paddock was breathing normally, correct?"

"Correct."

"You don't remember a code being called or have any recollection of what you were told at the time. Correct?"

"Correct."

"You don't know when you wrote the 2:20 P.M. entry saying that you had called the chief neurosurgery resident, correct?"

"Correct."

"You don't recall any of these details, but you definitely recall that Dr. Laws was never in the NCCU during the hours of 1:00 P.M. and 2:00 P.M. You definitely remember that. Correct?"

"That is correct."

Gary looked visibly disgusted, but he continued his onslaught.

"Nurse Boston. Referring back to the vital signs you took on Miss Paddock when she first arrived in the NCCU, one of those vital signs was Ms. Paddock's blood pressure (BP). Correct?"

"Correct."

"When Ms. Paddock first came out of recovery, her BP was 110/60. Correct?"

"Correct."

"And at noon, it had gone up to 140/84. Correct?"

"Correct."

"Correct me if I'm wrong, Miss Boston, but doesn't that constitute a widening pulse pressure and isn't *that* one of the signs of ICP?"

"I believe it is. Yes."

"You *believe* it is?"

"It is. Yes."

"Now we don't really know what her blood pressure had risen to by 1:00 P.M., because all we have are checkmarks indicating there was no change in her neurological status, correct?"

"That is correct."

"And you don't know what her blood pressure was at 2:00 P.M. because you didn't check her at 2:00 P.M., did you?"

"No."

"When you *did* finally check her at 2:20 P.M., her blood pressure was 158/82, wasn't it?"

"Yes."

"And you were supposed to call a doctor if her blood pressure had risen above 160. In fact the BP monitor would have sounded an alarm if the BP had risen above 160. Isn't that correct?"

"Yes."

"Nurse Boston. The chief neurosurgery resident in charge was a Dr. Kelly. Yes?"

"If that's what the records indicate, then I assume that is correct."

"Well, according to your own testimony given today, you were to notify Dr. Kelly if Miss Paddock's BP rose above 160 or dropped below 100. Isn't that what you testified to?"

"I believe so. Yes."

"And so you didn't think it was necessary to call Dr. Kelly when Miss Paddock's BP rose to 158, just two points shy of when the alarm would have sounded?"

"No. It wasn't over 160 yet."

"It wasn't over 160 yet?" Gary asked in disbelief. "It was just two points shy, but because it wasn't over 160 yet, you didn't see any cause for alarm?"

"In retrospect, I guess that was a wrong decision on my part."

"Oh my God," I thought, yet again. It was all I could do not to leap out of my chair and strangle her.

The cross examination continued.

"Nurse Boston, regarding the medications you administered to Miss Paddock. "You told Mr. Nash that you had given Miss Paddock thirty milligrams of codeine for pain."

"That is what I said."

"Is it possible you gave her more than thirty milligrams? Perhaps sixty milligrams?"

"No."

"All right. To the best of your recollection, what was the nature of the pain?"

"I remember it as being abdominal in nature, which is normal for that kind of surgery."

"You were aware that she had been given thirty milligrams for pain at 10:30 A.M. and then another thirty milligrams at 12:20 P.M., shortly after arriving in the NCCU, were you not?"

"Yes I was."

"And it didn't raise any alarms that she needed additional pain medication less than two hours later when the prescription called for 'every four hours?'"

"No. Not really."

"Thank you, Nurse Boston. Just a few more questions." Gary studied his notes.

"Nurse Boston, you gave Ms. Paddock 200 milligrams of Tigan for nausea, did you not?"

"That is correct."

"And you were aware that there were specific instructions saying that a doctor was to be notified if Tigan was being administered, were you not?"

"I believe so, yes."

"But you didn't notify a doctor, did you?"

"No."

"Why not?"

Nurse Boston was silent.

Seeing the jugular exposed, Gary went in for the kill.

"Nurse Boston, I'd like to take you back to the moment when you returned from lunch. You returned from lunch, stood at the foot of Miss Paddock's bed, and watched her breathing, correct?"

"Correct."

"And you believed she was breathing normally, am I correct?"

"Yes."

"But you didn't walk around the bed and try to rouse Miss Paddock, did you?"

"No, I did not."

"And it would have been simple to do so, wouldn't it?"

"I suppose so."

"And it would have been simple to check her pupils, wouldn't it?"

"I suppose so."

"And you just didn't do it because she was stable, according to your check marks, an hour earlier," Gary's voice rose, "isn't that right?"

"Yes."

"And so instead of assessing Miss Paddock, you went over to the other patient and took vital signs and checked his blood sugar levels, right?"

"That's right."

"And that took about twenty minutes, correct?"

"Yes."

"So it was one hour and twenty minutes between the time you last assessed Miss Paddock – according to your check marks – and the time you assessed her after your lunch, correct?"

"That's correct."

"And when you finally turned to Miss Paddock, she was stuperous, was she not?"

"Yes."

"Her right pupil was five millimeters and sluggish and her left pupil was three millimeters and sluggish, correct?"

"Correct."

"But you didn't call a code blue, did you?"

"No. I called Dr. Kelly and told him I was having trouble arousing the patient."

"Did you do anything before Dr. Kelly arrived? Administer any life-saving procedures? Any intervention?"

"No. I just stood there and watched the patient."

What followed was a pregnant pause as Gary seemed to be looking over his notes and thinking about his next step. The pause was punctuated with barely audible sighs. Finally, Gary lifted his head and quickly glanced at the jury. "One final question, your honor."

"Nurse Boston, I'd like to return to your description of the instructional materials you received in preparation for your placement in the NCCU. You say you received some additional take-home materials, perhaps even classes, on the topic of neurosurgery. Correct?"

"That is correct."

"Surely they weren't training you to be a surgeon?!"

"No. Neurosurgery nursing."

"Do you mean neuroscience?"

"Yes. That's what I meant. Neuroscience nursing," she replied curtly.

"Whew. That's a relief. Glad we got that cleared up."

"Objection!"

"Withdrawn."

And with that, Gary concluded his cross of Nurse Boston. He had destroyed her as surely as if a half-ton bomb had landed right where she was sitting in the witness stand. It was clear that her testimony had had a devastating impact on the defense's case and probably had a lot to do with the fact that the case was ultimately settled.

The fifth and final most memorable part of the trial for me was the day that Dr. Laws was called to testify. I remember it was the Friday before Easter. Good Friday, April 14, 1995. Dr. Laws had come up for that one day from Charlottesville, Virginia where he was now the Chief of Neurosurgery at the University of Virginia hospital. It was a day I was eagerly anticipating. I knew that my lawyers had thoroughly explored the question of whether Dr. Laws, himself, had been negligent and had found no evidence that Dr. Laws had done anything wrong. But I *felt* that he had carelessly and callously squandered the trust I and my family had placed in him. I had no recollection of what Dr. Laws looked like, but I wanted to meet this man face to face, to look him in the eye and demand an explanation.

Dr. Laws was the only witness called to testify that day. His testimony began in the usual way, with a run-down of his credentials. He was presently a Professor of Neurology and Medicine at the University of Virginia. He did his undergraduate and graduate work in New York City and completed his residency in 1970 at Johns Hopkins University. He worked at the Mayo Clinic for fifteen years, moved to GWUMC as chair of Neurosurgery from 1987 to 1992. He had authored close to 200 articles and six books. While at GWUMC, he supervised twelve residents at a time as well as the chief resident and interns. The NCCU was set up under his guidance.

"Your honor. We move to qualify Dr. Laws as an expert witness."

"No objection as to causation only."

Brian Nash then proceeded to question his witness. However, what I remember most vividly was Gary's cross-examination.

"Dr. Laws, there has been some discussion concerning the issue of timing. Specifically, there is some issue as to when exactly the bleed should have been detected and what type of bleed it was – venous or arterial. Do you have any opinion on either of these issues?"

"In my opinion, it was an arterial bleed, which means it was a fast rate of bleed. Given the fast rate of bleed, the brain would have decompressed rapidly and it could be a matter of only ten to fifteen minutes before signs of increased cranial pressure would be visible. It is also highly probable that the 400 ccs of cerebral spinal fluid (CSF) that had built up in the ventricles could have been pushed out of the 1.5 millimeter hole created when the VP shunt was inserted."

"And how long would it have taken for that volume of CSF to be pushed out?"

"With the patient flat on her back, about ten to fifteen minutes."

"Oh, no!" I thought. "This isn't going well at all. What is Gary doing? This doctor is destroying all the good work Gary has done! The defendant is trying to make the case that the VP shunt was taking up the slack of the bleed and therefore slowing down the signs of brain decompression. Oh, God. Please Gary. Just get this witness off the stand." I sat in silence, my eyes pleading for Gary to read my mind.

But Gary couldn't hear me. He continued with his questioning.

"Dr. Laws, can you determine the probable rate of bleeding?"

"No, I can't."

"What about the site of the bleed?"

"No. It is impossible to tell."

"On the second operation, when they removed the blood clot, could you tell the site of the bleed?"

"No. I couldn't determine that."

"Dr. Laws, we have heard testimony that the bleeding started when the patient left the Operating Room. Do you think that is a possibility?"

"No, I disagree with that."

In my mind, I felt myself screaming at Gary, "What are you doing?", but my mouth wouldn't open. I only thought, "You've just destroyed our case!" I sat in utter despair. But suddenly, I see Gary and Marian, as well as the opposing counsel, approaching the bench to speak with the judge. Gary is holding a document in his hand. It is Dr. Law's deposition. The lawyers and the judge are conversing. It is clear Gary is agitated. They seem to be discussing something about Dr. Law's court room testimony not being in accordance with his deposition testimony. The judge is shaking her head. "Motion denied. Improper use of deposition testimony."

To this day, I don't know what the controversy was about, but I suspect it had to do with what type of bleed it was - arterial or venous. In his deposition, Dr. Laws had said that it was a venous bleed, but on the witness stand, he contended it was an arterial bleed. For unknown reasons, Dr. Laws had changed his mind.

As eventful as Dr. Law's testimony was, what happened immediately before Dr. Laws approached the witness stand came close to being a showstopper. I entered the courtroom that morning and sat behind my attorneys as usual. Gary turned around and asked me, "Did you say hello to Dr. Laws?"

"No, I haven't seen him. Is he here?"

"He's sitting right behind you," Gary replied, looking amazed at my response.

I turned and looked at the man seated behind me. I didn't just glance at him. I stared long and hard at him, my eyes piercing through his body, trying to see into his very soul, and scanning his entire face searching for something that would trigger a memory. He seemed to be a stocky man, not too tall, dark hair, a jovial face. There was no recognition. Nothing. I had absolutely no memory of this man seated behind me, the man who, in my opinion, had destroyed my entire life and all my career prospects. I didn't recognize him. The words I had spoken in my deposition rang hauntingly true at that moment: "I wouldn't know him if I ran over him."

As unexpected as that was - I had always thought that upon seeing Dr. Laws, my memory would be jogged - what was even more unexpected was my reaction to finally seeing him and realizing who this man was to me. As far as I was concerned, this man had destroyed my life and yet, here he was, sitting calmly, less than a few feet from me. My reaction was not only unexpected by me, but it was unanticipated by my parents and by my attorney. So much so, that if the Judge hadn't immediately cleared the courtroom and, additionally, if the jury had been in the courtroom at that moment, my case might well have been declared a mistrial.

I lost it. I completely, totally, lost all control of myself. I started crying hysterically, repeating over and over the fact that I didn't recognize this man. The scream I cried out was like a combination of the sound of a shrieking hyena and the cry of a crane. But it was worse than even that. It was the cry of someone whose pain had been buried deep inside her for five long years, years defined by 45-minute therapy appointments, physical therapy, occupational therapy, neurotherapy, psychotherapy, years of additional surgeries, of pain and humiliation, memories of the destruction of my deepest dreams, the dreams that Sigmund Freud had described a century earlier as the very essence of being alive, of life itself: the ability to love and to work. I believed in the very core of my being that Dr. Laws had been responsible for destroying those hopes and dreams. All of that pain was now erupting to the surface with an agonizing and terrifying scream.

In a flurry of activity, Gary sprang from his chair, helped me out of my chair and together with my parents carried me into the witness waiting room. Why did three people have to carry me out of the courtroom? Because when I'm under any kind of emotional distress, such as being fatigued, being embarrassed or self-conscious, or crying, my left leg doesn't operate at all. I am rendered unable to walk. In trying to understand this, it might help to think of the human brain as a large circuit board similar to what telephone operators use. There is a right, left, frontal and rear panel of the brain. Each panel controls a specific function of the brain. For example, the right frontal area controls movement, judgment and emotion. However, within the category of emotion, the process of telling a joke is served by the front right hemisphere while the process of hearing and interpreting the joke is controlled by the back right hemisphere. When a person has sustained an injury to the brain as I had, one or more panels is rendered non-functioning. The brain then rewires the functions previously controlled by the damaged panel, in my case movement, onto an existing, undamaged panel, emotion in my case. When the panel that controls emotion is called upon to actually do the job it has been set apart for, it can no longer take on the dual role of controlling movement. And thus, I was rendered unable to move.

April 16: The night before the trial ended

I remember going to bed the night before the trial was scheduled to end with an overwhelming sense of doom. Actually I was filled with many emotions all intertwined in my mind and my soul: doom, despair, disbelief. In my untrained, inexpert mind the trial had not gone well for my side. I began to agree with the defense experts, who had said that if my depression could possibly be alleviated, my problems with fatigue, my memory problems - which are a direct result of fatigue - and a wide variety of emotional issues that I was dealing with would, in turn, be alleviated. So, I went to bed that night thinking our side was going to lose this case and how completely unfair that was, because I truly had been injured.

My life as I knew it and my career as I had planned it was now irrevocably over. The following scenario kept playing over and over in my head: I had accumulated $480,000 in medical bills and $35,000 in student loans. Physically, I would probably never be able to hold a full-time job, but in order to pay off all my loans, pay my rent, and support myself, I would have to have a full-time job. I envisioned a life of working fifty to sixty hours a week, working myself to exhaustion every day, coming home at the end of every day and collapsing, and never being able to go out and enjoy the company of friends, because I was either working or sleeping. In short, I would have no life outside of working to support myself. I would never be able to afford to buy a house, to drive a car, or experience being a twenty-something young woman again. I walked with a leg brace and a cane. I was elderly at thirty-two. I would never be able to save for retirement and would be a pauper if I ever did retire. My parents would be long-gone. My future looked as bleak as a desert, with no oases in sight. The testimony of my own witnesses made it clear that my life was as good as over. My nightmare would never end.

And so I laid down that night, put my hands together and decided to pray. I cannot explain why I thought prayer would work or that God would be listening to me. I could not remember praying as a child except for saying grace, perfunctorily, before family meals and the pro forma prayers at bedtime. In my mind, nothing much ever came of those prayers, but that night, with the trial about to end the following day, I felt I didn't have much to lose. And so I prayed. It was a short prayer. I beseeched God for an amount of money that I thought I could live with. In retrospect, it was an unreasonably small amount, given everything that my parents and I had endured (what attorneys call "pain and suffering") and given the years of unearned income I was facing (what attorneys refer to as economic damages) and given the fact that if I were to only work part-time for the rest of my life, whatever the jury awarded me would have to last me for the rest of my life, some fifty years, assuming I lived until I was eighty-two. Even so, that was the amount I prayed for. I fell into a deep sleep and waited for the next day to dawn.

Proceedings of last day: April 17, 1995

The presentation of the evidence came to a close and the judge adjourned the proceedings to give both sides a chance to prepare their closing arguments. My parents and I sat outside of the courtroom, talking. Gary was near us, by himself. The next thing I knew, he grabbed my arm and took me to the side.

"They have made an offer of settlement," he tells me. "However, before you accept it, there are some things I think you need to consider."

"What's the offer?" I asked.

He tells me. My heart leaps. It is the exact amount for which I had prayed to God the night before.

"Gary," I replied. "I don't need to think about it. I know you'll think this is crazy, but this is the exact amount I asked God to grant me last night before I went to bed."

"Well, you should have asked for more. I've seen the look on those jurors' faces. I think I can get you a lot more. You need to think about the medical bills you are going to have to pay in the future, not only the ones you have already accrued." Now that seemed like a reasoned counterargument and my parents agreed, so I told him, "See if you can negotiate more."

"I'll go back to them, but I doubt they'll agree. Not without a jury award. And then the Hospital will probably appeal."

"How long will that take?"

"No telling. It could take years. Do you want to seek Jack's advice on this?"

Jack was Jack Olender, the dean of medical malpractice lawyers in Washington, D. C. It was his firm that was representing me. "Maybe I *should* ask his advice," I thought. "He obviously has enormous experience in these matters."

So Gary contacted Jack Olender and he met us outside the courtroom. Gary explained to Jack that the defense had made an offer and that I was inclined to accept it. Jack asked me how I felt about it. I told him, looking up at him with my moist blue eyes, "Of course I'd like more, but I'm not willing to risk the appeals process and more importantly," I told him, "the award is the exact amount I prayed to God for last night before I went to bed."

"Well then," Jack Olender replied, "you should take it." Still not wanting to let go until all the "t's" were crossed and "i's" dotted, we agreed to wait until Gary had a chance to speak with Blue Cross/Blue Shield and confirm whether they would reduce their lien on the amount of the award I might get. They agreed. And it was done. We accepted the settlement offer. It was over. And I could now get on with the next phase of my life.

I had no idea what the next phase of my life would entail, but I did feel that I had achieved closure that Tuesday afternoon in April 1995, after five debilitating, excruciating, grueling and agonizing years. The highly experienced attorney for the Hospital could read the jurors' faces as well as we could and he could see that the jurors had concluded that I was worthy of their compassion and their generosity under the law. In my view, I had won. And more importantly for my life after the trial, I believed with all my mind and all my heart that my prayers had been answered.

3

The Hospital: Where It All Began

"And I could now get on with the next phase of my life, whatever that may be." It's funny how when the totality of one's life is too much to deal with, a person tends to break down life's major events into stages. There were certainly many stages on my road to recovery, starting with my three months at The George Washington University Medical Center (GWUMC). As part of my research for this book, I tracked down many of the health care specialists who had treated me at GWUMC. This was important for me for two reasons. One, I wanted to thank them and show them how all their efforts paid off. Secondly, since I had no memory of my stay there, I was hoping to recapture time, put faces to names that my parents had mentioned, and trigger some kind of memories.

Actually, to say that I have no memory of my stay at GWUMC is not completely true. What I *do* have are a few brief images, visions as it were: people or moments that echo in my mind. I sometimes remember faces that are encircled in a gray cloud, similar to an old black and white photo.

For example, I remember sucking on the cotton swabs that had been dipped in various-tasting liquids. According to my mother, the purpose of these swabs had been to keep me hydrated, but the flavored swabs were also intended to reengage the swallowing mechanism of my brain and to stimulate the muscles of my mouth.

SEARCHING FOR THE OPEN DOOR

I also have a memory of sitting in a chair, most likely a wheelchair, with a pen in my hand and a large, black woman leaning over me. I appear to be sitting at a desk. My mother says this memory is of the time when the hospital's social worker was helping me to sign a power of attorney over to my parents. Since my writing hand was my left hand and the entire left side of my body was completely paralyzed, I can only imagine what a long, drawn-out ordeal that must have been.

I also discussed with my mother another vision I had of my sitting on an airport runway in my wheelchair and watching a plane take off. She couldn't even imagine what memory that could be connected to. All she could guess was that this corresponded to the time when my aunt, who lived on the outskirts of Crozet, Virginia, had come to visit me on her way to England. Somehow, my subconscious was aware of the reasons my aunt was there and my brain retained an impression of me sitting on the runway and watching her take off. I believe it is more likely that this image was how my brain explained and interpreted the fiasco surrounding my discharge from GWUMC.

These three images fall into the category of weird or amusing, but there is one memory I have that haunts me to this day and for which no one has come up with an explanation. My parents came to the hospital every day and stayed with me from noontime until I was put to bed, roughly at 8:00 P.M. They bought many audio books-on-tape and would leave the tape playing when they departed the hospital for the evening. Their intention was for the voice on the tape to soothe me, to keep me company, and to keep my mind engaged when they could not be at my bedside to talk with me themselves.

However, one night as I was listening to a tape, I heard all sorts of loud banging, doors slamming and people yelling down the hallway. A real sense of fear spread through me and I attempted to make myself as small as possible, to slink down into my bed and hide under the covers. I hoped and prayed they wouldn't come for me. The next day, I remember asking the day nurses what the loud noises had been. No one knew, or would say, anything about it. To this day, it remains a mystery to me. The fear I felt that night was brought on by my sense of complete helplessness. Here I was, at the mercy of anyone and everyone who wanted to come in and do me harm. I couldn't walk, I couldn't run. I couldn't even get out of bed. All I could do was scream.

These dim, vague "memories" aside, I still wanted to find some of the people who had treated me at GWUMC in order to capture some of the *details* of my stay there. Of all the GWUMC health care providers I managed to find and visit when I sought them out twelve years after my discharge in August, 1990, none was more genuinely thrilled and surprised to see me than Julie Ries.

Julie Ries was the physical therapist who had treated me at GWUMC. She is a slightly-built woman, about 5'7" tall with blonde hair. She was twenty-six at the time of my accident, the exact age I was. She apparently re-marked to my parents several times, "She's the same age as I am. I've just got to help her." And so she did, staying late afterwards to work with me, holding me longer for therapy and even coming in on weekends occasionally. I went to see Julie in her office on August 21, 2002. She had moved to Marymount University, just outside of Washington, D.C. in northern Virginia.

"Oh, my God. I can't believe it! You look so *great*! And your *arm*! How in the world did they straighten your arm out?" And that was the beginning. The rest of the visit was an exhilarating ride upward from there. I asked her to look through the medical records I had in my possession, which detailed some of the therapy I was given while at GWUMC but which I couldn't decipher, either because of the handwriting or because it was a poor copy.

As she sat down with me, I examined the reaction she was having as she read the words on the pages. Her facial expressions ran the gamut from consternation - as she remembered how ill I had been - to delight, as she glanced at my now-smiling face.

"Wow!" Julie exclaimed. "As a therapist, I would see patients like you on a regular basis in the hospital, but once the patient is transferred to rehabilitation, you lose track of them. Unless the patient tries to contact the therapist some time in the future, you just never know how people end up. I just can't tell you how phenomenal it is to be reading your medical record and having you sitting here in front of me: alert, verbal, oriented, lucid. Incredible!" Julie's elation still echoes in my mind to this day. I strongly urge any person who has made significant progress through therapy to seek out their former therapists. It not only helps them as the patient to appreciate how much they have achieved, but it also provides encouragement to the therapist to see the fruits of their labor.

Julie's memories of me when I was in the Intensive Care Unit (ICU) were much more vivid than her memories of me at other times. What she remembered most was my arm and the process she went through in trying to figure out what to do about it. My left arm, as you may recall from the trial testimony, had ended up at about a twenty degree angle to my body, with my elbow turned tightly into my chest. It was a completely useless and non-functioning limb, as was my left hand, my writing hand.

"I can't remember if we decided we couldn't do the serial casting of your arm until we had done a muscle block on it to allow us to pull your arm outward. Your arm was so flexed that you had skin on skin, the inside of your elbow was overlapped onto the skin over your left forearm and bicep. For hygiene purposes we couldn't try to put your arm in a cast, because your skin would break down from sweat. We were working so hard to get your elbow to straighten. You were at full flexion. Your arm couldn't have been any more bent."

I sat right next to her as she read through the chart, looked into her eyes and asked, "As you read through the record what do you see? What in particular leaps out at you?"

"I can see how low-level you were early on in terms of being able to participate. The record I'm looking at right now starts on June 8, 1990. You were one-month post-op. You were still very sleepy, nauseous, and vomiting a lot, probably from all the medication you were on. We tried to use bright objects and tactile objects to stimulate you, but we were completely unsuccessful.

"This record is dated the middle of June. It was then that you began to break out of the persistent semivegetative state you were in. You began responding to your environment, following basic commands. There's a note in here that says, 'responsive only to painful stimulation'." Seeing me wince, she paused. "I know that sounds awful, like we were torturing you or something, but you must look at it from a medical perspective. If you have a patient who is not interacting with his or her environment at all, you need to see if there is a connection, if the brain is even functioning. Your only option is to try first some sort of noxious-type stimulation, like a pinch or a bad smell in the hopes of eliciting a response. If that doesn't work, then you have to resort to more painful types of stimulation. You have to do this, or the insurance company will throw the patient out, having determined that there is nothing more that can be done for you. All the insurance company sees at this point is that you are taking up a bed that someone else might need and costing them money.

"You were dangerously close to the time when the insurance company was going to refuse to pay anymore, to 'pull the plug,' as we say. I remember that we were doing everything we could do to keep you there. When day after day, the progress notes indicate 'Patient unable to participate. No real change,' the hospital is hard pressed to make a case for why you need to stay. Especially in this day and age, under managed care, if there is no change in a patient's status for a couple of days, then it is hard to justify continued therapy. It was much easier in the early 1990s to do what we were doing with you—that is to keep trying to stimulate you on a daily basis in the hopes of breaking through. You have to continually reevaluate and reassess. But you really don't know what is and what isn't helping the patient."

She looked troubled as she continued her assessment of the deplorable state of the health care system. "Because of all the changes in health care, insurance companies will refuse to pay for services that they conclude are not having any benefit. Now, what we end up doing is educating the family and creating support networks to try to maintain what we have done already. In 1990, when you were in the hospital, I could still go in and perform passive range of motion therapy on you, because it was considered a form of physical therapy. I would not be permitted to do that today. It is not considered a skilled service. *Anyone* can give you passive therapy. But who is to say that the interaction you and I had didn't facilitate your eventual recovery? In 1990, if there was no change in status, I could just keep coming back. Today, if I saw you for two or three days and you were not responding, you couldn't be aroused, and there was no change in that period of three days, then I would not be able to justify continuing to have you on my physical therapy schedule."

A shudder went down my spine as I realized the implications of Julie's statement. "What you are saying is that if what happened to me in 1990 had happened to me today, I could very well still be a vegetable."

"Yes. If you come away with anything from this experience, it is an increased awareness of how important it is, today, for caretakers of a newly-disabled person to take the time to find medical professionals who know how to work within the rules and are able to provide others with training on how to care for the patient. Something like performing passive range of motion therapy is easy to learn and, as your case illustrates, this seemingly unimportant therapy is extremely vital in the scheme of things."

She continued reading the progress notes.

"There was a gap in therapy, according to the therapy notes. There is a note written on July 6 and July 9 and then nothing until July 16. You apparently had developed a fever, so we were unable to do therapy for a week. According to the notes, therapy finally resumed on July 16.

"Wow!" she exclaimed, hurriedly flipping through the pages. "This is incredible. As I read through these notes, I can see you coming alive with each passing day. On July 16, all of a sudden you became responsive: you were waving hello and goodbye. You repeated my name on request. You participated in a twenty minute therapy session in which you demonstrated active head rotation and could perform reaching moves. You exhibited the ability to brush your own teeth. You still couldn't tie your own shoelaces, however. I believe it was at this point we attempted to move you into the regular physical therapy department instead of performing therapy at your bedside.

"On July 17, the record indicates you came to the physical therapy department for the first time. You tolerated a one-hour session with frequent rest breaks. You were definitely plagued by inordinate sleepiness the whole time you were at the hospital. I suspect this was a combination of the medication you were on and the fact that you had gone from being in a reclining position during your coma to being upright. At this point in your therapy, our emphasis was on head and trunk control. You didn't have the neck strength to hold your head up so it was bobbing around like a rag doll. We had to place a collar around your neck to keep your neck upright and to redevelop your neck muscles."

"I remember that!" I exclaimed. "Actually, I have memories of wearing that collar at Magee Rehabilitation Hospital (Magee) in Philadelphia. I think I had entered the 'terrible twos' at that point and kept ripping it off my neck and throwing it on the floor."

She laughed.

"The progress notes show a substantial improvement in your level of alertness over the next three weeks. Your head control increased. You were able to rotate your body to the right and flex and extend your arm a little. The notes indicate that we worked on you being able to roll to the left side."

"Like a baby."

"Yes. A baby learns to roll before learning to walk. I remember it was harder for you to roll to the right, because in order to do that you needed strength on the left side which you lacked, because of the paralysis on the left side of your body."

"What else?"

"Well, at this point we were up to one-hour sessions, with less frequent rest periods needed. Our main emphasis appeared to be on mobility training, sitting activities, and head control. In the beginning, you required maximum assistance to remain upright when sitting on the edge of the bed, which means the therapist was doing seventy-five percent of the work."

Being overwhelmed by the realization of how far I had to work my way back, I attempted to change the subject slightly and focus on the notes pertaining to the speech therapist. This was by far the most interesting of the therapies I underwent and I have often thought about going back to school and studying to become a speech therapist myself. I have come to learn over time that the term "speech therapist" is somewhat of a misnomer. A speech therapist *does* focus on speech in the case of a patient who has a speech impediment from birth, a stroke, or some other ailment. However, in *my* case, the speech therapist worked on a multitude of other issues, primarily cognitive in nature—such as memory and sequencing—but also issues pertaining to the interaction between the brain and the muscles of the mouth, such as the ability to swallow. I remember swallowing being a huge problem for me, my parents and my caretakers, because it meant my nutrition was coming from liquids rather than solid foods. That situation can have all sorts of repercussions on the health and movement of one's bowels. A feeding tube had been inserted into my stomach early in my hospital stay and, one month later, it was still there. In fact, I was dependent on the feeding tube until well after I had arrived at my next rehabilitation stop, Magee in Philadelphia.

According to the progress notes that Julie could decipher, my speech therapist evaluated me for the first time on June 6th, and then reevaluated me six weeks later, on July 19th. At that time, she found me to be alert but tired. She had significant difficulty maintaining my attention and focus. Today, I am certain that I would have been diagnosed with attention deficit disorder or ADD and put on a medication to treat it. Apparently, I did know my name, where I was and what year it was. The speech therapist noted an increase in the strength of my oral motor muscles, but remarked that I was still drooling heavily. I remember having the drooling problem well into my stay at Magee. In fact, I still wake up on occasion with drool on my pillow or notice that I have been drooling slightly when sitting watching TV or reading a book. I find it embarrassing.

My memory and my inability to retain focus were of great concern to the speech therapist. She noted in her progress notes that I had trouble completing commands, "not because she can't do it, but because by the time she gets around to doing it, she has forgotten what she is supposed to be doing."

Julie continued her reading of the progress notes.

"You started to become more verbal and you were obviously in a lot of pain for some reason," she comments.

"How do you know that?"

"Well there is a notation in here that 'you have been moaning a lot today.'"

"What else?"

"Well, you began to answer selective questions, but you seemed to get lost in thought between the question and your answer to the question."

"Why was that, do you think?"

"I suppose it had to do with your ability to process new information. That ability had definitely been impaired by your injury. Someone would tell you something and it took you a while to formulate an appropriate response, if you ever did respond. It says here that you needed constant coaxing, but that you were responding to verbal commands, such as eat, do this, don't do that."

Growing weary and depressed by hearing Julie interpret the barrage of notes describing my condition, I attempted to redirect Julie's attention to a happier aspect of my rehabilitation – my attempts to learn to walk again.

"Let's focus back on the notes from the physical therapist. What do they say?"

"Well, you are now able to lean to the left to maintain your balance, but only when someone tells you to do it, known as 'cueing'. You had severe limitations in your elbow and shoulder, brought on by the way that your arm ended up after the surgery. I've noted here that I can see improvement in your ability to sit and maintain your head upright."

She continued her reading of the notes.

"You appear to have been getting more and more frustrated with the physical therapy as time went on. That's probably because you were becoming aware that you were unable to do many of the things that had never been hard for you before your surgery. I imagine that *would* be frustrating," she said with a smile, glancing kindly at me. "I remember you were a very bright girl before the injury," she said.

"Yes, I was."

"Well, you still are. I'd wager that, even with your diminished brain capacity, you are still brighter than the average person out there."

"Now here's something interesting," she remarked. "There is a note written on July 23 by the occupational therapist. It says you were seen again by an occupational therapist for a splint check of your left foot due to your constant movement and alertness. Apparently, you were able to remove the foot splint on your own and would do so if it was hurting you."

She laughed. "Looks like the neck collar wasn't the only thing you hated wearing. Actually, the fact that the brace was uncomfortable and you were proactive in doing something about it was a good sign."

"I don't remember the foot splint," I told her. "All I remember was being fitted at Magee for a huge cast on my left leg, which I had to wear 24/7, even to bed."

"Well, that cast was probably the replacement for the foot splint. You were wearing the splint at GWUMC, because your left ankle was stiff and prone to foot drop. If that hadn't been corrected, you would never have been able to stand with both feet level on the ground. This would have meant you would never have been able to walk, because your left foot would have been frozen on a diagonal to the floor. It says here in the progress notes that the doctors expected the foot drop on the left side to resolve itself once you began to put weight on your legs, because the foot drop on your right foot had resolved itself. But that didn't happen with your left foot."

She continued reading. "The July 24 entry notes that you were put on the tilt table for the first time."

"The tilt table?" I asked, having never heard of this device.

"A tilt table looks a lot like the stretcher that they use to wheel patients to surgery. They place you on the table to begin the process of weight bearing. They place you at increasing angles to the floor and hold you in that spot. They are trying to get your muscles strengthened in your leg, hip and abdominal region to support the weight of your body when standing. It is a more gentle and gradual way to get a patient upright."

"Go on."

"There is an entry here on July 25. 'Seen for forty-five minutes in speech therapist's office. Continuing to address memory problems. Patient now has delayed recall with seventy-five percent accuracy. Patient able to decode single words and large print. Positive gag reflex. Decreased cues required.' Well those are all encouraging," Julie said.

"I guess. I still have a real problem with my short-term memory. It is very frustrating to my family, my boss, my husband and me."

"You'll probably struggle with that for the rest of your life. Try not to be so hard on yourself. I see from these notes that the occupational therapist was still trying to get your swallowing mechanism to engage."

"How do you know that?"

"There is a notation here: 'Still has weakness in the muscles around the mouth, creating fluid pockets, because the muscles that hold the form of the mouth can't maintain the fluid in there.' "In other words," she smiled, "you were drooling. The occupational therapist recommended a video swallow test to determine exactly which mechanisms were working and which were not. "

"What does the fact that I was drooling have to do with swallowing?"

"Well, all day long we are swallowing our saliva. So if your swallowing mechanism is not working, the only place for the saliva to go is out through the mouth. Your brain is the CPU (central processing unit) of your whole body. When a part of the brain is damaged, it will affect whichever part of the body was dependant upon that part of the brain to operate. In this case, because your windpipe and stomach are linked through the same pipe, if your brain doesn't know to block off the windpipe when you swallow, you will choke."

She continued reading the notes. "Emphasis on sitting activities. Your sitting balance is improving. You are able to maintain a sitting position for seven seconds with supervision. That is terrific progress. Just one week earlier, you required maximum assistance and now you can sit there with someone sitting beside you for up to seven seconds. Your head and trunk control has also improved in just one week's time."

She stopped, a puzzled expression her face.

"Now that's weird. There is a discharge summary dated July 26, but you weren't actually discharged until August 12, almost three weeks later. Hmmm."

"Well, perhaps this time *I* can shed some light on what happened," I said. "I affectionately refer to this incident as the discharge fiasco. The insurance company finally pulled the plug and ordered the hospital to discharge me. They thought I was being discharged on July 27. I was due to be transferred to St. John Medical Center (St. Johns) in Tulsa, Oklahoma where my parents lived and where I grew up. However, the receiving doctor called my parents that day and informed them that St. Johns wouldn't accept me, because I was too close to going into rehabilitation and there was no rehabilitation clause in my student health insurance policy. They basically didn't want to get stuck with me, without any assurance of getting paid."

"So what happened?"

"Well, my parents first offered to pay for the rehabilitation themselves, knowing it would probably bankrupt them. My mother had stopped working at that point and, and at the age of seventy, my father was due to retire soon. If my parents had gone forward with their intention to pay for the rehabilitation regardless of the cost, one of them would have had to go back to work. They were advised against doing this and so, as a last resort, they telephoned the Associate Dean of Students, George L. Crowell, at The Johns Hopkins School of Advanced International Studies (SAIS), where I had been a student, and he put the large gears of the Johns Hopkins bureaucracy into motion."

"What do you mean by that?"

"Representing the University, George Crowell approached the student health care insurance representative to see if there was anything he could do. The man Dean Crowell consulted, Sam Shriver, was a godsend. He didn't even know me, but he went to bat with Blue Cross/Blue Shield of Maryland and got them to insert a managed care/rehabilitation clause into the student policy retroactively. It was truly a miracle. This opened the door for a case manager to investigate the facilities of the various rehabilitation centers around Washington and determine which facility would be best for me. They ultimately decided on Magee. I wouldn't be here in the shape I am if that hadn't happened."

"I'll say. Sounds like your parents really came through for you."

"Both they and Dean Crowell of SAIS. I cannot stress enough how important it is for the person, who is providing care, to be proactive about getting the rehabilitation the patient needs if they want to ensure the patient recovers as much as possible. My parents pulling out the stops and getting Johns Hopkins to spring into action on my behalf was instrumental in my recovery."

Julie paused again and looked at me. "You look tired. Shall we stop?"

"Well, how much do we have left to go?"

"Only the last three weeks before you were finally discharged."

"Well, okay, let's finish this up then."

"You made remarkable gains the last three weeks you were at GWUMC, although you flunked your video swallow. You aspirated some liquid that you were given."

"What were the gains?" I asked. I think I must have sounded a little annoyed. What I was thinking was, "What in the world is wrong with me? I must really be an idiot. I can't even manage to swallow like a normal person. Swallowing! For goodness sake, how hard can that be?" Little did I know that if I thought swallowing was challenging, learning to tie my shoes again would be entering a whole new universe of difficulty.

"Well, in early August, they began serial casting your arm in an attempt to straighten it out. August 2 was your first cast and they managed to get you to ninety degrees, which was enough to avoid the skin-on-skin problem."

"What does serial casting entail?"

"Serial casting is when they inject some kind of solution into the muscles of the arm to relax the muscle so that you can then reposition the arm. You cast the arm in the new position and keep it there for about a week. You continue this process until the arm is fully straightened.

As I said, they managed to do this until you at least didn't have the skin on skin problem."

"What other progress was made?"

"Well, you were still incontinent during physical therapy and had to interrupt your therapy on occasion to change your underwear."

"Yes, I remember that. My life since the brain injury has been one embarrassing moment after another."

"Well, you must learn to focus on the positives. By the time you left GWUMC, you had reached the point where you were able to sit upright in and propel a narrow, lightweight wheelchair. You were also able to transfer from the bed or chair to the wheelchair with moderate assistance. Your balance when sitting was static. The note says, 'fair at best with tendency to fall backwards.' Head control was a fair minus. By August 3, a week before your release, there is a note that says, 'substantial gains'."

"Regarding your memory skills, the occupational therapist noted that you recalled a paragraph with eighty-five percent accuracy. That means that your memory was improving. Your ability to process information was also improving. She notes that you could discuss the pros and cons of a given scenario within thirty seconds with close to seventy-five percent accuracy."

"Gee. I was becoming a regular genius."

"Stop it," she scolded me. "Those were substantial improvements given where you had started.

"In physical therapy, you were starting to move your left upper extremity. Your active movement had improved and you could move within full synergy patterns. You could extend every joint at once or flex every joint at once, but couldn't isolate a particular area or joint. This is one of the biggest problems with neurological insults. We haven't yet figured out how to get the brain to send a more specific message to the muscle or the extremity, individually. And that's about it, except for the discharge summary. You were transferred to Magee on August 13, 1990."

4

Magee Rehabilitation Hospital:
Learning to stand before you can walk

Anyone who has spent time battling the intransigence and medical ignorance rampant in American insurance companies in order to receive the care they, or a loved one, requires will appreciate my own struggle with insurance companies. Suffice it to say, if it hadn't been for my parents' dogged determination and tenacity, I would never have gotten the rehabilitation I needed. I have been particularly blessed in my life by having extraordinarily loving, devoted and heroic parents. Both my parents were willing to sacrifice everything to make sure I had every therapy I needed to make as complete a recovery as possible so that I could rejoin society as a functioning human being.

After my parents, Sam Shriver and George Crowell had successfully lobbied to get a rehabilitation clause inserted into my student medical policy, I was transferred to Magee Rehabilitation Hospital (Magee) in Philadelphia on August 13, 1990. My discharge summary from The George Washington University Medical Center (GWUMC) constituted a roadmap of where I had been, and where I still had to go before my rehabilitation could be considered complete.

As I entered Magee, cognitively, I was able to follow one and two-step commands in therapy, although with a significant delay in my responses. I remember very clearly when I was at Magee trying to participate in a conversation. It was like trying to carry on a conversation

Magee Rehabilitation Hospital

in an Internet chat room. There was a noticeable delay between the question being asked and my response, as my brain tried to make sense of what was being asked and to formulate an appropriate response to the question. On that topic, the speech therapist noted in my discharge summary from GWUMC that my verbalizations and responses to questions were appropriate, when I ultimately made any response at all.

There is a notation that I scored 20/30 on my neuropsychological evaluation. I was later told that that score corresponded to about a fifth grade level of intellectual ability. I definitely remember those tests. I took four of them during my six-month course of therapy at Magee and my later rehabilitation program at PATE Rehabilitation Endeavors, Inc. (PATE) in Dallas, Texas. They were grueling all-day tests, seeking to measure one's ability to perform in every area of the brain: spatial acuity, mathematical, verbal, logic and reasoning skills, time sequencing, writing, speaking, and memory.

Another progress report from my discharge summary emphasized my inability to form words the way I wanted to, because of the lack of strength in my muscles in my mouth and the lack of motor skills. As my mother had said in her deposition, I was truly like a baby and apparently, I talked like one as well.

In terms of my auditory and comprehension skills, the discharge summary noted that I could answer "yes or no" questions with 100% accuracy. Answering abstract questions were far more difficult for me. I had great trouble focusing my attention. I needed constant repetition and constant refocusing on the task before me. I could identify objects with 100% accuracy, but I was unable to identify which object did not belong in a group of similar objects. At that point in my recovery, I did not perceive that a banana did not belong in the same group with a baseball, a cap and a mitt. The concepts of categories, items that were parts of wholes and analogies were completely lost on me.

My mother later told me of another test with shapes that were cut out of a piece of tile - a square, a circle, a star, and a rectangle. I was unable to discern that the square lying next to the piece of tile should be placed in the part of the tile that had a form cut out of it that corresponded with the square. Six months later, I was able to complete these seemingly simple tasks, principally because my mother and father did not give up and they, in turn, would not let me give up. And no one facing a similar situation should give up, nor should those who love them and are caring for them.

My verbal expressions, although syntactically correct, were few and far between and I only spoke if I was prompted to do so. In addition, compared to my pre-surgery voice, which I have now regained entirely, the volume of my voice was weak and I had a very flat affect, meaning that I had no intonation or facial expressions. This was the "dawn of the dead" look about which my mother had testified during the trial. I spoke very much like a robot.

My memory deficits continued to plague me throughout therapy and, indeed, continue to this day. If I read a paragraph, I was barely able to recall important details even two minutes later. Five minutes later, it was as if I had never read the paragraph in the first place. This did not bode well for a student still hoping to return to her graduate studies. I also suffered from enormous fatigue throughout my two-year course of therapy. This, too, would be a significant challenge for a graduate student. This fatigue further hampered my recovery to the point that my afternoon therapy sessions were often unproductive. I remember my mother alluded to this in her deposition taken before the trial. "She would sleep a great deal. She would have to nap in the morning and nap again in the afternoon. I mean a good long nap."

In terms of my physical condition, I had moderate to severe limitations in my left shoulder and left arm and hand in terms of my range of motion. This also applied to my left foot and ankle, which was almost frozen in a downward position. My ability to right myself was inconsistent. If someone started to push me over, there was a fifty-fifty chance I could bring myself back to vertical without assistance. I could sit up and roll with minimal assistance. However, I still needed a great deal of help to transfer myself to a wheelchair, to squat, and to turn. My left ankle remained extremely unstable. It still remains unstable and I continue to walk with an ankle brace full-time.

I remember laughing when I read the part of the discharge summary concerning my eyesight and whether my ability to see, my visual acuity, had been compromised by the operation. The reason I found this comical is because someone on the GWUMC hospital staff had misplaced my glasses while I was in physical therapy. I had vision of 20/700. I could not see a darn thing without glasses. Of course I had visual deficits. All they had to do, I kept telling them, was find my glasses and I'd be fine.

However, a successful performance on the swallow test continued to remain beyond my reach. I was still being fed through a tube when I left GWUMC. I finally learned to swallow again about two weeks into my program at Magee. That success made possible the removal of the feeding tube and I was able to eat solid foods at last. I had entered GWUMC at a weight of 130 pounds. By the time I left the hospital, I was *still* five feet five inches tall, but I only weighed eighty-nine pounds.

Magee took over where GWUMC had left off. The doctor in charge of the brain unit at Magee was a respected physiatrist named Dr. Lawrence J. Horn. A physiatrist is a physician who specializes in restoring optimal function to people with injuries to the muscles, bones, tissues, and nervous system through the practice of physical medicine and rehabilitation. Dr. Horn tried a then-novel technique known as muscle blocking, which involved injecting the muscles that had too much tone in them – in my case the gastrocnemius soleus complex muscle in my left calf, which was causing my foot to point downward. This block essentially deadened the muscles so that they could no longer impede the recovery of my other muscles. This technique when coupled with serial casting, as was performed at GWUMC, helped minimize my foot drop. This enabled me to put both feet on the floor and, eventually, to walk upright.

Dr. Horn also attempted to take up where GWUMC had left off and serial cast my left arm for a second time, using muscle blocks as he had done with my left foot. This time he focused on the bicep and extensor muscles of my left arm. This treatment was a success. The process straightened my left arm from a twenty degree angle to my body to about an eighty-five degree angle to my body. Over the course of the next ten months after I was discharged from Magee, my mother, who had been taught at Magee, engaged in daily, excruciatingly painful exercises with me during which she had to stretch my tendons and muscles that had shortened. She was determined her child would not end up a cripple. I remember screaming, crying and yelling at my mother to stop when the pain became too much for me.

"Do you want to walk around with your arm like this for the rest of your life, never having any use of it?" she asked me.

"Yes. I do. I don't care any more. Please just stop!" I screamed.

But my mother refused to stop and through her determination, she was able, eventually, to straighten my arm to almost a 180 degree angle to my body.

The sense of helplessness I had experienced that frighteningly noisy night at GWUMC grew more intense upon my transfer to Magee, mainly because I was becoming more aware of my surroundings and of my own impaired physical condition. Anyone who has been a patient in a hospital is familiar with the loss of one's sense of self: one is no longer a person, but rather a nameplate, a disease, a diagnosis. The skimpy gowns one must wear deprive each patient of his or her dignity. If you are lucky, a kind nurse will show some compassion. Unfortunately, especially today, with the ratio of nurses to patients growing larger and larger, many nurses are simply too busy to show any compassion. They have a job to do. Moreover, thanks to the litigious society we live in, there is also no room for going outside of prescribed rules and norms and going the extra mile.

A good example of this is the way Magee handled the issue of my missing glasses. At the time I arrived at Magee, I was totally unaware of the fact that my glasses had been lost at GWUMC and of the fact that I was therefore unable to see, because I was unaware of my surroundings in general. However, with my increasing general awareness came an increasing awareness of how helpless and dependent I was, as well as how visually-impaired I was without my glasses. I remember sobbing uncontrollably over meals because I was unable to see what I was eating. One friend of mine from Philadelphia, who was visiting me, tried to console me by saying, "Trust me, Cynthia. You don't *want* to see what you are eating!"

One weekend my aunt came from New York City to visit me. I started telling her about my glasses having been misplaced and how frustrating it was for me.

"Here, try mine, she said." I put them on.

"Oh my God. I can see! Oh, can I have them, please?" I begged her.

"Well, I need these, but I've got an extra pair at home. I'll send them down to you right away."

She pulled them away. I sat in my wheelchair, grasping for them, like a child seeing her favorite toy being ripped from her hands.

True to her word, Aunt Phebe sent her second pair of glasses to me via Fed Ex. With glee, I ripped the package open, knowing what was inside. I immediately put them on. I was ecstatic. How marvelous it was. I could see! No longer would I be isolated in my room while my roommate and a nurse watched "America's Funniest Home Videos," wondering what they were laughing at.

Unfortunately, my joy was short-lived. One of the nurses saw me wearing the glasses.

"Oh, so they finally found your glasses!"

"No," I answered tersely. "These are my aunt's glasses. She had an extra pair."

"Do you have the same prescription?"

"Nearly," I lied. There was no way in hell they were taking these away from me.

"Well, you can't wear them. You've got an eye doctor's appointment scheduled in a few weeks, and we want to have a true and accurate baseline assessment of your visual deficits." And with that, I was relegated to the world of gray, blurry images yet again.

The sense of helplessness and frustration brought on by this incident was repeated later in my stay, this time with my contact lenses. The check up with the eye doctor revealed no lasting impairments in my vision. He even suggested I try using my contact lenses again, which my mother had been faithfully cleaning and storing for the past five months. However, since I didn't have any fine muscle control in my fingers, I was unable to put the contacts in myself. So, I had to rely on the one nurse who was brave enough to put them in for me. When that nurse wasn't there, I was out of luck.

All these incidents combined highlight one of the main problems with being in a hospital or rehabilitation setting. Not only do you have to contend with the fact that you are not well, but you also have to contend with the overwhelming sense of helplessness and powerlessness you feel as your world is spinning out of control. In short, you suffer a complete loss of independence. This loss of independence becomes more acute, the more you become aware of your surroundings. Becoming more aware of your surroundings has its upside and its downside. On the one hand, when people reach the point at which they are aware of their situation, they can easily begin to despair about their condition. However, that is not the time to despair. It is the time to become even more motivated. By becoming so acutely aware of their loss of independence, people are, in fact, developing the powers of reason and thought to do something about regaining their independence: they are now reaching the point where they can fight their way back and win.

Losing one's independence can be especially traumatic if you are confined to a wheelchair. If I learned anything from this overall experience, I learned patience. For example, I have had to wait for people to help me and wait while everyone else got off the plane, even at the risk of missing my connecting flight. In the rehabilitation hospital, I had to wait for someone to open the door for me so I could push my wheelchair down the hallway to the dining room. I also had to rely on someone to get me to the bathroom in time. Couple that with my brain's inability to "signal" me before the very moment when I have to go and I am lucky to get to the toilet in time. I remember several times when I was in a wheelchair that I was unable to do so. It was humiliating. It was even more humiliating when I was incontinent even though I had enough time to get to the toilet, because the wheelchair wouldn't fit through the bathroom doors. The problem of incontinence has been an ongoing issue for me, occurring even as late as 2003, while I was at work. The terrible problem of incontinence goes far beyond the physical discomfort and embarrassment: it affects the psyche and self-esteem of anyone who experiences it, whether the person is twenty-six years old or seventy-six years old.

I left Magee on October 18, 1990, almost nine weeks after I arrived. On paper, the discharge summary from Magee does not appear significantly different from the discharge summary from GWUMC. In fact, however, I had made substantial gains, in both the physical and emotional realms, although the cognitive areas were still lacking.

Physically, with Dr. Horn's successful intervention, I was able to plant both feet level on the ground. As my muscles grew stronger, I was able to progress out of a wheelchair. By the time I left Magee, I was walking with the help of a quad cane, the kind with four "feet". In order to walk, you must have the cane planted firmly on the ground, which makes walking much slower, but decidedly more steady, and for anyone who has trouble maintaining their balance, infinitely safer. With the quad cane, I could walk about sixty to 100 feet at a time, under constant supervision. I continued to be dependent on my wheelchair for longer distances. Magee graciously loaned us a wheelchair upon my dismissal, with the proviso that we had to return it when I no longer needed it. I was able to stand for up to eight minutes to perform basic self-care in the morning and evening, such as washing my face and brushing my teeth. However, I still had trouble with my balance. Specifically, I didn't know where my midsection was in space. I didn't know how to stand erect and so, to avoid falling over, I needed someone to tell me to shift my upper body to the left or the right, whatever the case may have been.

Emotionally, my increased awareness of my surroundings and my situation led to a very real sense of my enormous helplessness and dependency on everyone around me, especially my parents. I developed a condition my parents fondly refer to as the "Niagara Falls" syndrome. Visiting hours were at 4:00 P.M, every day and my parents would come like clockwork every day at that time to see me. At a few minutes before 4:00 P.M., I would wheel my wheelchair out of my room into the hallway and plant myself firmly by the doors they were expected to come through. Someone had mistakenly given me a watch as part of my rehabilitation therapy, in order to teach me to tell time again. I say "mistakenly," because I sat there at the doors of the locked brain injury ward and waited, looking at my watch. If my parents were even *one minute late*, I started sobbing hysterically. Actually, my parents say it was closer to the sound that an injured wild animal makes. The brain injury unit was located on the fourth floor of the hospital. My parents tell me they could hear me wailing as they stepped onto the elevator on the ground floor. The wailing continued as they made their way up the four flights, rounded the corner and then approached the hallway where the locked, double doors were located. This condition prompted Dr. Horn to add one more medication to my already long list – Prozac. He claims he did it for the benefit of the other patients and the staff. Whatever his reasons, I couldn't wait to rid myself of it. The remedy worked. I stopped crying incessantly. Unfortunately,

Magee Rehabilitation Hospital

Prozac worked too well. It rendered me completely emotionless. I did not cry or laugh. I hated it.

In terms of activities of daily living or ADL, I was able to independently dress myself as long as my shirt had no buttons. I needed only slight assistance to put on my bra, underwear and pants. I could prepare a cold sandwich also with minimal assistance. However, how to tie my shoes remained a mystery to me and I was still in diapers. Along with toilet training, learning to tie one's shoes is another activity that is a lot harder for a twenty-six year-old to accomplish than it is for a three year-old.

I finally passed the swallow test and was weaned off of the feeding tube over the remaining course of my stay at Magee. Having entered Magee at just eighty-nine pounds, the goal then became to break the 100 pound threshold. The staff at Magee poured every conceivable food item down me. I remember receiving menus every day with a wide array of foods from which I could choose, and I could choose as much as I wanted, as long as I ate everything I selected. For me, this was frustrating. I had never been a big eater, and now I was being forced to gorge myself and yet my weight never seemed to increase. I know. We all wish we had that problem. Magee couldn't release me until I broke the 100 pound threshold. They tried everything, including supplementing my diet with a high-calorie, vitamin-rich drink.

The nurses called these drinks fortishakes. I hated them. They gave me one at lunch and another one at dinner. I could not leave the table until I finished it. You would have thought they had given me a whole plate of brussel sprouts to eat the way I labored over this fortishake. I thought it tasted terrible. I would literally throw temper tantrums over being forced to drink it. I came to find out much later that the only problem with them is that the staff had served them to me warm, which is why they didn't taste good. I discovered this upon my return to Washington, D. C. when I again was having trouble with my weight. I kept seeing these commercials about a high-calorie, vitamin-rich drink and so decided to try one. Much to my surprise, they were fortishakes and when chilled, they were delicious. It is funny how things come full circle.

The inclusion of the fortishake into my diet did the trick. I passed the 100 pound threshold and was released from Magee a week later, on October 18, 1990. I came to learn later that I was discharged none too soon since the insurance company again was balking at paying for any further hospitalization. In fact, I was later to learn that Dr. Horn had managed to keep me there two weeks longer than the insurance company wanted by asserting that there was some new treatment he wanted to try on me.

I remember my release from Magee as if it were yesterday. During this time, I was consumed by the feeling that I was the central figure in a horrible nightmare and that I would awaken at any moment. My parents picked me up in the Plymouth Voyager they had purchased during the two weeks when they had gone home to Tulsa after my admission to Magee. We drove to Virginia to see my father's sister-in-law, who lived outside Charlottesville. I remember my mother waking me up in the middle of the night to take me to the bathroom (part of the toilet training process) and my being completely disoriented. I thought I was still at Magee. I kept telling her to be quiet

Magee Rehabilitation Hospital

because we'd wake up the other patients. On another occasion during that same visit, I was afraid to go into the bathroom, because I thought somebody was in there. It was not until we turned into the driveway of our home in Tulsa, Oklahoma that reality set in. This was not a nightmare. It was my new life.

5

PATE and Kaiser Rehabilitation programs:
The End of the Rehabilitation Road

With my departure from Magee Rehabilitation Hospital (Magee) in Philadelphia, and my return to my parent's home in Tulsa, the continuation of my rehabilitation was again in doubt. For the second time, Blue Cross/Blue Shield refused to pay for any additional rehabilitation. I was functioning at a basic level and that was all the insurance company's decision-makers believed was necessary. What did it matter to them that I still had the mind of a child? What did it matter to them that, although I had one year of graduate work completed and spoke two languages, all I was equipped to do was perform a menial job at a fast food restaurant? My mother, my father, and I all prayed that the insurance company would agree to give me the type of cognitive rehabilitation that I so desperately needed at that point.

With the insurance company refusing to pay anymore, my mother became my primary caretaker. As she said in her deposition, "I literally devoted two years of my life to this kid's rehabilitation. I was determined that she would not regress while we were waiting to get her into some other type of rehabilitation program." According to my mother, I was very much like a baby when I left Magee. The staff had gotten me as far as they could physically, but mentally, I still had the abilities of a toddler. Magee had given my mother some materials to use to try to help develop my ability to think. In addition to a variety of exercises designed to strengthen my memory, there were exercises in which I had to compare a series of pictures and determine which objects in the picture were alike and which were not.

My mother and I also concentrated on strengthening the fine motor muscles of my left hand so that I could write again. While at Magee, I had been using my right hand to write, and not very successfully, since I had always been left-handed. I remember being given a thick pencil with which to write. It took me so long to write just one sentence with my left hand that, out of frustration, I would change hands and start writing with my right hand. I've often joked that I should have been a doctor, because my handwriting when using my right hand was that bad.

I remember fondly one particular aspect of my therapy during my three-month time in Tulsa: the jigsaw puzzle. My best friend in Tulsa was Laurie Winslow; we had been childhood friends. We were next-door neighbors growing up and only two months apart in age. Her composure upon seeing me for the first time since the injury was impressive. The gentleness she displayed as she came over to my house and patiently helped me put a jigsaw puzzle together is a testimony to her character. It must have been traumatic for her to see her friend barely able to walk and in diapers. However, she later told me that it was not until she sat down with me to complete the jigsaw puzzle that she truly grasped the extent of my injury. I kept trying to put pieces together that obviously had no relation to each other, either because they didn't match in color or size or didn't correspond to the area of the puzzle we were working on. I was not even able to understand that the straight edge pieces were the border of the puzzle. Looking back, I can smile when I think about it. At the time, my reaction to my inability to participate in an activity enjoyed by young children was one of humiliation: I felt ashamed, ill at ease, and just plain stupid.

Just as I began to spiral into a depression, a door opened. Blue Cross/Blue Shield agreed to further rehabilitation and I was sent to Dallas in January 1991 and enrolled in the program sponsored by the Greenery Rehabilitation Center. My parents were overjoyed. Time is of the essence when dealing with a brain injury. If cognitive therapy does not begin soon after the injury occurs – usually within one year of the injury is considered the window of time—there is a chance that some cognitive aspects will be lost forever. As far as I am concerned, even though I have made a remarkable recovery, that four-month lapse in cognitive therapy has had lasting effects.

The Greenery Rehabilitation program had two parts. The first was a ranch, which served as an independent living facility. There I learned to dress myself, keep time, and cook simple meals. I also continued with physical therapy. On February 13, 1991, after six weeks at Brinlee Creek Ranch, I entered the cognitive portion of the program, which took place at a facility just outside of Dallas, Texas. This program was run by PATE Rehabilitation Endeavors, Inc. and was designed to be a day program only. I was placed in a suite at The Embassy Suites hotel and continued doing Activities of Daily Living (ADL) to further myself along the path of returning to a normal life. However, the main focus of the program was cognitive recovery, where my deficiencies were most significant. Without more cognitive recovery, my hopes of returning to my graduate program at The Johns Hopkins School of Advanced International Studies (SAIS) would never be realized.

The discharge summary from Magee detailed the main problem areas in my cognitive rehabilitation. I had severe attention deficits and moderate-to-severe functional memory deficits. I was now at a twelfth grade reading level, up from the fifth grade reading level I had shortly following the brain injury but down from the graduate reading level I had before the injury. My reading comprehension was also moderately impaired. I had trouble processing information and coming up with the appropriate responses to questions. I had difficulties in planning and organization, time management, reasoning and judgment, attention to detail and endurance. In terms of my behavior, I was still very much like a child. Simple problems appeared catastrophic, my emotional reaction would be dramatic, and only after I calmed down was I able to reason through to a solution. At the top of the agenda was redeveloping my interpersonal skills and teaching me techniques to manage my responses to stress.

The cognitive therapy at PATE consisted mostly of coursework. Since my ultimate goal was to return to graduate studies, the therapists focused on simulating a classroom setting for me, complete with lectures and exams. Unfortunately, they got off on the wrong foot by choosing psychology as the subject. That choice made sense from their perspective, because they were all trained psychologists. However, I was extremely bored reading the textbook and took every opportunity to tell them so. Having shown myself to be very opinionated, if not uncooperative, they relented and one of the psychotherapists agreed to teach a course in economics. For me, this was another mistake. Now my pride took over. "What in the world," I thought, "could this man teach me about international economics? I was a graduate student at SAIS." In retrospect, I am ashamed of my ungrateful attitude and my behavior towards the psychotherapists, who were just trying to do their job and help me on the road to recovery. If I could, I would apologize to them in person. Having gone through several years of psychotherapy, I now understand what was at the root of this behavior. By this time in my recovery, I had become keenly aware of how much brain damage I had actually sustained. Concepts that had once come easily to me were now hard for me to grasp. My attitude was a reflection of the frustration I felt upon realizing this. Effectively, I tried to build up my self esteem by tearing down the psychotherapists.

During the final week of April, the staff at PATE called my parents in Tulsa to inform them that the insurance company had cut me off and that my parents should come to Dallas and take me home. This came as a complete shock. I had only been in the cognitive program since February 13, a little over two months. My parents had expected that I would be able to continue with this therapy through the end of May. There had even been treatment plans devised that carried therapy through until the end of August! My parents pleaded with the insurance company, impressing upon them how important it was for me to continue with the cognitive therapy. But the insurance company refused to pay another cent.

And so, on May 2, 1991, my parents packed up my belongings and drove the five hours back to Tulsa. They had been driving down to see me every weekend since I had started at the Ranch. Now, they would be driving back to Tulsa for the last time. "We were at a loss as to what to do," my mother said in her deposition. "We finally got in touch with the director of the program at PATE, who told us to get in touch with Dr. Terry Shaw." Dr. Shaw, as you may recall, was the first neuropsychologist to testify at my trial. He was based in McAlester, Oklahoma, about an hour and forty minutes from Tulsa, but he worked part-time at Hillcrest Hospital in Tulsa, specifically in the Kaiser Rehabilitation program at Hillcrest.

Dr. Shaw suggested contacting the Oklahoma Department of Human Services to see whether I qualified for free admission into the day program at Kaiser. With my assets near zero, I was definitely qualified, financially. But would they take me? Was I too far along or not far enough along? That was the question.

As far as I was concerned, all this was irrelevant to my world. For my part, I saw my goal of returning to graduate school by the fall of 1991 slowly slipping beyond my grasp and that was all I cared about. I tried to console myself. "What did it really matter *when* I returned," I told myself. "All of my classmates would already have graduated from the two-year master's degree program in which I had been enrolled. All my friends were gone. I'd be starting over anyway." Still, the thought of staying another year in Tulsa, Oklahoma seemed unbearable. Other than my next door neighbor, I did not have any friends

PATE and Kaiser Rehabilitation programs

left in Tulsa. "Miserable," I thought. "It will simply be miserable."

My parents' valiant, last-ditch effort to secure further rehabilitation through the State of Oklahoma system was successful. I entered Kaiser Rehabilitation in Tulsa seven months later, in December 1991. The primary focus at Kaiser was on strengthening my arms and legs and increasing my endurance. I was also given more physical therapy outside Kaiser. However, with no direct cognitive therapy, the danger that I would begin to plateau intellectually and in terms of my memory was very real. And along with that, my dream of returning to graduate school in Washington was slipping ever further away.

During the seven-month wait for the State's decision regarding funding for further rehabilitation, I enrolled in a marketing course at the local junior college in the fall of 1991. This was to prepare myself for an eventual return to my graduate program. It was also the only way my parents could think of to counteract the effect of the sudden discontinuation of my cognitive therapy. The marketing course was followed by a course in accounting in the spring of 1992. I then went to San Antonio, where my oldest sister, Susan, lived and enrolled in Accounting II at the community college there that summer. Having me enroll in the second semester of Accounting at a school away from home was a brilliant move on my parents' part. It removed me from their constant supervision, placed me in a more independent setting, and further put me on a successful path that would lead to my return to Washington, D. C.

I came through the three courses with flying colors, achieving a grade of A in each one. But I wondered whether community college level courses would prepare me for the world of highly competitive, over-achievers in Washington? Always looking out for my interests, my mother and father referred the decision about my ability to return to graduate school to an expert. Dr. Terry Shaw, who had administered the previous tests, administered yet another neuropsychological evaluation in May, 1992.

To prepare for writing about my long path to recovery, I recently listened to the tape that was made at the May 1992 meeting with Dr. Shaw, my parents and me to discuss the results of his testing. What is most striking about that tape is how differently my parents and I interpreted the results. As far as I was concerned, Dr. Shaw had told me that most of my deficits had been reversed and that, with the use of a few "compensatory" techniques, my cognitive condition was good enough to resume my graduate studies. My parents interpreted the results quite differently. They thought resuming my graduate program was premature. My mother cited the fact that I had to work harder at things that had come easy for me before the injury, such as writing. "She used to be an extremely good writer, but I've noticed that her organizational skills are not what they used to be," she said in her deposition. Drawing attention to issues such as my verbal attention problems and the fact that I am easily diverted, she voiced her concern about whether I could make the return to SAIS successfully and if I failed, how this would affect me. As is usual, the truth of the matter lay somewhere in between those two interpretations of the data.

While citing the continued deficits of memory, visual processing and visual learning, Dr. Shaw responded, "You don't have deficits as much as you have relative weaknesses, your left arm and leg are the most obvious of these. Your dexterity on your left side is still slower than your right side. However, you have learned to compensate extremely well."

He continued, in that kind, gentle – almost fatherly - tone of voice to which I had grown accustomed. "Your visual processing system is not as efficient as before. This directly impacts your ability to navigate social situations."

"Why is that?" I asked.

"Well, that's because the law of socialization is not verbal. It is visual. Therefore, you will likely be prone to misread social cues and facial expressions. You'll be constantly having to ask someone, 'Are you angry with me?' for example. In addition, because the little voice inside you that says, "Don't say that." isn't working as it should, you risk saying things that people will find offensive or will take the wrong way. It will take a lot of understanding on the part of others for you to be able to successfully surmount these difficulties and avoid alienating friends and co-workers.

"Another difficulty you will most likely have is in the area of time management. You are prone to underestimate the time it will take to complete a task. This is because you are having to operate in a world that you know, but with a different set of tools than you had previously. You have trouble organizing things in proper sequence to make the most efficient use of time. You have learned the benefits of writing out a schedule as one compensatory technique to counter this problem.

"Most importantly as it relates to going back to school: your memory deficits. Your delayed memory, working memory, and retention were severely impaired by the injury. And your memory is still not back in the range it was prior to your brain injury. This means you can't cram like you did before. You have to approach your study around one hour time blocks. Any longer than that and your brain will begin to shut down from receiving too much stimuli at one time."

As his remarks and observations sunk in and I felt myself sinking under the weight of all the hard work ahead of me, he offered up a piece of encouragement and a few more words of fatherly advice.

"You'll do fine," he said. "It'll be more difficult, no doubt. But the old techniques will still work for you. I know you have some concern about economics. Economics was difficult for you before. Will it be impossible now? Well, that depends on your attitude. Put your pride on hold. Don't be ashamed to get a tutor or a study partner if you need it. Don't discount your ability to overcome the difficulties you are having. I know what you are thinking and going through. You've had people messing with your life for two years. Now you want to be back in control. But you have to be realistic and ask for what you need. Don't let your pride take away your chance to succeed. You've had to swallow a lot of pride in the past two years. What's the big deal about losing a little more pride?

"Going back to school and succeeding is not a measure of your self worth. Your self worth has been already established. Be less interested in how you look when you are climbing the mountain. Be interested in reaching the top even if someone has to push your butt up the mountain from behind."

PATE and Kaiser Rehabilitation programs

That piece of fatherly advice from Dr. Shaw has become my mantra. It is a great mantra for anyone, who finds themselves in such a position or who is caring for someone in a condition such as mine. I have found this advice to be applicable to any disabled person, because it goes to the very heart of recognizing that you can still achieve your goals in life, but you will need to learn how to ask others to help you get there.

6

August 1992–May 1994: Back to the Beginning

In the end, my desire to return to The Johns Hopkins School of Advanced International Studies (SAIS) and finish my degree prevailed over my mother's objections and concerns. And so, at the end of August 1992, we packed the car and drove to Washington, D.C. from Tulsa.

I remember my return to SAIS as if it were yesterday. All my work in therapy and my hopes and dreams for two difficult years had focused on that day. I had looked forward to this moment for two years. It was what had kept me going through all the painful, and at times incessantly tedious, therapy. And yet the moment had finally come. Was I ready? Or were my parents correct and it was still too soon? I had accomplished so much and believed I was now up to this challenge, but what would it be like to return to graduate school after two years? All my friends with whom I had been in school had already graduated. How would I manage without the camaraderie of my classmates who had been there with me in 1989? I was pretty sure that I would make new friends, but I was so different now. I was older, almost six years older than most of my classmates. And I was disabled. I stood out not only physically but mentally as well. I felt out of sync. Friendless. Lost. Dr. Shaw's parting words, "there's a good chance you'll be self-conscious going back" were ringing in my ears. And then, all my fears and embarrassment of walking into the school with a brace on one leg and a cane in one hand suddenly vanished. Just inside the doors to the main entrance stood a young woman, clearly a student. She walked up to me as I entered. I'm sure I looked as confused and hesitant and out-of-place as I felt.

"Are you Cynthia?"

"Yes."

"Welcome. I'm Ladan Archin, student body president. We've been expecting you." And with that, I embarked on the next phase of my life. I didn't know where it would lead me, but I knew I was going to meet it head on.

In retrospect, returning to SAIS and attempting to reenter the world outside of hospitals, rehabilitation centers and the warmth and love of my parents' home was even more difficult than I could ever have imagined. I felt so different. In attempting to interact socially, I was directly confronted by the reality of my new situation. In 1989, I used to gather with other students at the weekly Friday night "happy hour," move on to dinner, stay up half the night at a party, then wake up the next day to do my homework. Now, I could no longer drink, because liquor further impaired my ability to walk. I could not party until the wee hours of the morning, because I was still plagued by fatigue, sleeping at least nine hours each night and requiring a nap every afternoon.

Studying was now a full-time job, because I had so much to do just to keep up with the pace of even one course. I took a small tape recorder to each class; taped the two-hour lecture, and then spent another two hours transcribing my notes. Sometimes I even paid students who were already taking the class to take notes for me. I hired a tutor for my economics and financial analysis courses. The SAIS administration gave me extra time to

take my exams, because my left hand – my writing hand
– was still weak. I also received extended time in which to
turn in the class writing assignments, beyond the normal
grace period accorded other students. I also took a re-
duced course load, only three classes, down from the
requisite four that the other students took. And I enrolled
in no language instruction until the following summer.
Throughout all this, I was still allowed to retain my
fellowship, despite the fellowship's requirement that I
take a full course load of four courses, thanks to the
kindness and flexibility of the Associate Dean of Students,
George L. Crowell.

But my greatest challenge was the reduction of my
cognitive abilities, which had been the subject of so much
expert testimony at my trial, because these were hidden
from the sight of everyone I met. I had to learn how to
interact with fellow students, teachers, and potential
colleagues, fully cognizant of my "hidden" deficits and the
effect they might have on each and every one of my
interactions. Once again, help came from another SAIS
student, Sylvie Bossoutrot. Standing 5'4" tall with a wide
face and big eyes, Sylvie was a petite, attractive and
bright little blonde. As her last name suggests, Sylvie was
from France, although she was also half-Croatian. I think
it is the Croatian half that dominates her personality, at
least in her dealings with me. At the time, she lived three
floors below me in the apartment building across the
street from SAIS. I met her as she was walking along the
sixth-floor hallway, holding a lamp in one hand and
muttering to herself. We bonded almost immediately. I'm
not sure why exactly, but I think it had something to do
with her grandmother. She told me I reminded her of her

grandmother. For my part, I was drawn to her by her kindness and her innate interpersonal skills, skills I sorely lacked because of my brain injury. She accepted me as I was, and never made me feel as if I were different. She helped me integrate myself back into society and helped me immensely in regaining my self-confidence when it came to my course work.

While at SAIS, Sylvie was my constant companion. We remain good friends to this day. She saw me through two breakups with boyfriends and another major brain surgery in December, 1993. She also helped me survive countless term-paper writing sessions, exams and oral exams. I can truly say that my return to SAIS and the transition back into real life would have been far more dramatic and far less smooth if Sylvie had not been part of it. And she was part of it all, including graduation.

Like my first day at SAIS in August 1992, I remember the glorious day when I graduated from SAIS as if it were yesterday. It was May 26, 1994. I was so excited. This was my brass ring. I had done it. It had taken me four years, but I had defied the odds, surmounted the obstacles, and achieved my one, constant goal throughout four grueling, exhausting years. I was thirty years old, and I was graduating. I remember it was a beautiful, warm, sunny day. There wasn't a cloud in the sky. My graduation class descended the long staircase, walked across the courtyard and entered the church where the graduation ceremony would take place. Already my leg was acting up out of nervousness. My ankle would try to turn over and I was using all my strength to keep it stable so that I would remain upright.

I sat among my classmates, listening to the class speaker, listening to the keynote speaker, watching as individual students walked in front of the stage to receive various awards and then finally it came time for the Associate Dean of Students to hand out the diplomas. We started to form our lines as we had rehearsed the day before. The first to be called for his diploma had been the last to walk into the auditorium and therefore was sitting in the first seat of the first row. Row by row we stood up, went up to the front and waited to hear each of our names read aloud. Dean Crowell was at the podium.

I had rehearsed this moment in my mind dozens of times. I had told Dean Crowell that I wanted a hug from him when it came my turn. The name of the student ahead of me was called and he moved forward across the stage. My whole body was shaking with a combination of anticipation, excitement and fear. I was afraid that my leg might give me trouble as I started to walk across the floor. Dean Crowell handed the diploma to the student just before me and then paused. Looking straight into my eyes, he smiled and said with great authority in his voice, "Cynthia Paddock". I began to walk slowly across the floor. To my great relief, my leg was not causing me too much trouble. And then it happened. I heard a deafening roar. It was so loud I remember that I actually started to duck. I didn't know what all the commotion was about. And then my leg, as I had feared it might, started to go into a spasm and I found myself dragging my left foot behind me across the stage, making my journey to the podium even slower. Dean Crowell stepped off the po- dium to give me a hug. Tears began streaming down my face. I turned to look at the audience. They were all on

Back to the Beginning

their feet, clapping wildly. They were giving me a standing ovation. I couldn't find my parents in the sea of faces, but I found Sylvie and went over to where she was sitting and gave her a hug. Clutching my diploma in one hand and my cane in the other, I had fulfilled my dream. Despite all the obstacles, I had fought back from a complete and total vegetative state, from months in a wheelchair, learning how to swallow, to sit, to stand, to walk and to regain my memory and I had now earned my master's degree in International Relations.

The next day, however, I sat in my apartment feeling extremely let down. My fifteen minutes of fame were over. I had accomplished this great achievement, but now what? What did the future hold for me? I had graduated, but I had no job. Few of my classmates had jobs, but it would be harder for me to find one. Having concentrated in my studies on learning about the former Soviet Union and yet unable to travel extensively to that part of the world, what were the chances I would ever get a job in my field? Doubts were everywhere and I wondered why God, if there was a God, would have brought me so close to my dream, only to strip it all away. Once again, I found myself looking ahead to the next chapter of my life, with no idea of what it would hold.

7

The Gap Between Prediction and Reality

It is now July 4, 2007. As I sit in my home office, gazing out at the canal that runs behind our Fort Lauderdale home and watching the tall masts on the sailboats docked across the way as they sway in almost perfect harmony on the river, I cannot help but be in a state of constant astonishment at the almost complete transformation of my life and of myself since that ill-fated surgery seventeen years ago. I look back at not only the injuries and the physical challenges of overcoming the medical malpractice to which I was subjected, but also at the hurt, sadness and lost hopes that had to be resolved and, ultimately, redirected into a new and positive understanding of my life. I can now appreciate that my reality, although not everything I had once hoped it would be, is a life that is truly a good life, especially when contrasted with what it was predicted to be by the experts.

I could have opened up my own pharmacy with the list of medications I was on when I left Magee Rehabilitation Hospital (Magee). I was taking tegretol to treat my seizures, prozac for depression, dantrium to treat the tone and spasticity in my left arm, probanthine in an effort to strengthen my bladder control, Ampicillin to treat infections, and Desquam gel 5% to treat my acne. Sixteen years later, I'm down to none. Zero medications.

Contrary to the opinion of the expert witnesses at the trial, I did get married. The fact that I am married runs counter to all the expert testimony of the difficulty I would have with interpersonal relationships because of

The Gap Between Prediction and Reality

my inability to read body language, facial expressions, and correctly to assess vocal intonations. All the visual cues needed to successfully interact with another person do not play a significant part in my marriage. My husband is a very successful attorney, five years my senior, who became completely blind at the age of fifteen. He and I have learned to communicate with each other verbally, which, fortunately, was the one area of my brain that was not permanently impaired.

The bleak future I had envisioned the night before the case was to go to the jury also did not come to pass. Thanks in large part to the settlement I received, with which I made wise investments, and to the fact that I married a man with stable income, I am not living paycheck to paycheck as I had feared. I have been able to pay off my student loans and, together, my husband and I have achieved the American dream of owning a nice car and a nice home.

However, the experts *were* correct in their assessment of my career prospects. After a brief attempt to continue along my career path, it became quickly apparent that I would be unable to work a job that required long hours and a great deal of travel. Nor could I handle a job that entailed a lot of stress and required me to interact with people in unstructured situations. Moreover, as my neuropsychologist Dr. Terry Shaw predicted, I was constantly bumping up against the difference between what my resume showed I was qualified to do, and what I was actually able to accomplish, given my cognitive and physical impairments. My once-promising career in the Russian field was unrealized. I became so depressed that I contemplated suicide on more than one occasion. Driving such thoughts, of course, were the difficulties I encountered in interpersonal relationships and the realization that all I had worked for and the one goal that had kept me going during rehabilitation – my desire to return to my studies and continue along the career path I had set for myself – was now no longer a dream I could achieve. I had reached my goal of returning to my graduate studies and completing my degree, but in the end, working within my field proved impractical.

"I contemplated suicide on more than one occasion." And yet I did not end my life. I have lived to see many more days and countless truly happy days. Why? Is there an explanation? How, I have asked myself, does one explain my recovery against all the many doctors' predictions? Luck? Luck had something to do with it. The support of family and friends? Certainly few people have been blessed with a greater mother or father than I. Their dogged determination to ensure I received the rehabilitation I needed, and my mother's determination, in particular, to make sure my left arm was straightened out, were instrumental in my recovery. A successful lawsuit? Indeed, the settlement certainly took the edge off of what would otherwise have been a precarious and uncertain financial future. I have been able to continue with therapy when insurance companies have refused to pay, and to take advantage of new, more expensive technological improvements as they have become available. However, I continued to wonder whether there was something more? Was there something inside of me or outside of me that made it possible for me to pick myself up by the bootstraps and go on with life? My search for the answers to these questions was a long process that resulted for me in

The Gap Between Prediction and Reality

a renewed awareness and acceptance of the existence of God. At some point, I concluded that a greater force exists that makes believing in the impossible, possible.

Oddly enough, until I had gone through all my rehabilitation and examined the results, I had never thought very much about God. Of course, I had prayed for a positive outcome of the trial, but that was more of an eleventh-hour effort to do something, anything, to affect the outcome of a process over which I had no control. I did not pray from a specific belief in the power of prayer or in God's ability to answer prayer. If truth be told, although I was born and raised in the Bible Belt and was taken to church by my parents, I never really knew what it meant to be walking in God's footsteps. On the outside I appeared to be God's little angel – sweet and smiling - but inside a deep-seated anger was growing within me and I became a very angry teenager. I remember once I walked up to a neighborhood boy with my hands cupped and told him I had captured a beetle. I asked him if he wanted to see it. As he eagerly buried his face in my cupped hands, I threw the handful of sand I was holding into his eyes. That was terrible. What makes a young person do that? I remember another time when I tried to talk a friend into jumping off a ten-foot wall outside of the school. I claimed that I had done it and that she was just being a coward. Thank goodness her mother appeared and stopped us. I shudder to think what would have happened if my friend had acted on my dare.

I do not know what triggered my transformation from a sweet, angelic and obedient child into an adolescent full of anger and resentment, but I think the cause centered around the fact that my father was forced into early retirement from Shell Oil Company and, to make ends meet and provide us with a decent education, my mother had to go back to work. I was then ten years old and the only latchkey child on our upper-middle class block. Not having my mother at home was humiliating, not to mention lonely. That anger followed me into my college years where, free from parental oversight and guidance, I was able to act out that anger. That acting out invariably took the form of drinking myself into oblivion two or three nights a week and living a loose and carefree existence. Despite this dangerous behavior, I never ended up in the hospital with alcohol poisoning nor suffered the agony of being in a car accident. And so, in looking back, it seems to me that God's hand was at work even then protecting me from serious injury and or death. Many of my fellow co-eds, whose behavior was much like my own, were not quite as fortunate.

The anger that followed me into my college years was further exacerbated by my encounters with people whom I considered to be religious fundamentalists and judgmental. I could not then, and still cannot, tolerate the behavior and attitude of those types of individuals. To me, they are not so different from the Pharisees of Jesus' time, against whom Jesus continually railed. And so I turned my back on the church and religion entirely after I graduated from college in 1986. And then came May 7, 1990.

The events surrounding that tragic day, May 7, 1990 had a major impact on my life for it brought about a spiritual awakening. As bestselling author, Jim Stovall, accurately pointed out in an August 6, 2007 interview, "it takes a life-altering event to move from religion to relationship. " Jim Stovall further elaborated that "one's faith has to go from a theory that you take down and polish off on Sunday mornings to something real that you can live with."3 This is a statement with which I wholeheartedly agree.

When people experience any kind of misfortune, devastating disease, or loss, it is not unusual for them to end up bitter and angry. I certainly ended my whole ordeal that way. And I continued to be angry and bitter for years. Then, one Sunday, about a year after I was released from Magee, while I was in rehabilitation in San Antonio, I went to church with my sister, Susan, who lives there, and with whom I was staying. On that Sunday, the pastor delivered a sermon about a shepherd and one sheep that was always running off into the woods, getting lost or otherwise getting into mischief. After several failed attempts at discipline, the shepherd finally broke the sheep's legs and then carried him on his back until the sheep's legs healed. From that moment forward, the sheep never strayed far from his master's side. That sermon really spoke to me, because I felt that, in many respects, the story of that sheep was the story of my life. Hearing that parable was the beginning, I think, of my spiritual awakening, a process that has taken more than a decade of my life.

This spiritual awakening did not occur overnight. Upon returning to Washington, D.C. in 1992 to continue my graduate studies at The Johns Hopkins School of Advanced International Studies (SAIS), I started going to

---

3 Jim Stovall, Author of <u>The Ultimate Gift</u> in an August 6, 2007 interview with Maurice Broaddus.

church with a law school friend of my father's, more from a need to have some sort of social life than a need to commune with God. Nevertheless, it was during these weekly trips to church that my feelings began to change. The pastor at the church I was attending constantly preached the "Good News," the Gospel, and the fact that, as an example of the ultimate sacrifice and an example of all that a parent will do to save his child, God sent his only son to live on this earth as a human and to ultimately die for the sins of the whole world so that we mortals could be reconciled forever to Him. "Who was this God?" I asked. "Who was this God, who was so loving and self-sacrificing that he would do this? Was this the same God, who had left me paralyzed and in a coma and forced me to abandon my chosen career path? And what about the God who let six million Jews be murdered in the Holocaust? What kind of God was this?"

I came to understand that while I would never be able to answer all these questions, what I could do was to try to make sense of my own situation. And so I began to search for the meaning of my existence in an attempt to discover why I was literally saved from death. Did this God that I was hearing so much about have a plan for my life as the Old Testament of the Bible says in Jeremiah, Chapter 29, verse 11? "For I know the plans I have for you," declares the LORD, "plans to prosper you and not to harm you, plans to give you hope and a future." If so, what was it? In embarking upon this search, I tried to answer the questions: "How can a person enter the hospital for what is supposed to be a routine operation and end up paralyzed on the left side of her body, in a coma, unable to walk or talk, being fed through a tube, with the

The Gap Between Prediction and Reality

I.Q. of a vegetable?" And, "How is it that same person, whom doctors predicted would be in an institution for the rest of her life and unable to continue along her chosen career path, survive the odds and live to fight another day?" How indeed?

A scene from the movie, *The Sound of Music,* kept playing over and over in my mind. In this scene, Maria has run away from the Von Trapp family household and is seeking refuge in the convent from which she had come. The Mother Superior finally calls Maria to appear before her and asks why she had run away from the Von Trapps. "I don't really know," Maria replies. "I just couldn't bear seeing him anymore." It turns out that Maria has fallen in love with Captain Von Trapp and, out of fear of the unknown and because she had no experience in how to deal with such a situation, she fled. The Mother Superior says to Maria, "When God shuts a door. He almost always opens a window."

The phrase has always stuck in my mind and as I reflect on events in my past, I see how that phrase very clearly applies to my own life. As I examined the various turning points in my life: my ultimate choice of careers, my decision to leave New York and enter SAIS, the process by which I ended up at Magee, even the events surrounding my meeting my future husband, I began to see the possibility that there was a larger force in the universe at work, a greater Being who had a plan for my life and was constantly shaping events, leading me down a path to an ultimate, but as yet unknowable, goal.

The first turning point was my graduation from college. I graduated from Amherst College in 1986 with a B.A. in Russian Studies. At the time, the field of international relations was dominated by the Cold War between the United States and the Soviet Union. There were few jobs in the Russian field outside the defense or intelligence sectors. I knew I wanted to stay on the East Coast, principally because that was where most of my friends were going to be. So, after several months of searching for a job, I accepted the first one that was offered to me. It was at a commodities trading firm, located in Manhattan. I didn't have an especially good feeling about the job, but I accepted it anyway, because it enabled me to remain on the East Coast. I knew there wasn't a prayer of getting back to the East Coast if I were to return to Tulsa.

The job turned out to be an unmitigated disaster and I was fired just shy of my first three months, making me ineligible to collect unemployment. There I was, alone in New York City, with no friends, one aunt, no job and rent to pay. After a couple of days licking my wounds, I collected myself and went into an employment agency. They had a job on the books that they believed would be ideal for me. Unfortunately, the employer was already in the second stage of interviews. Nonetheless, the personnel manager agreed to see me. I interviewed for the job and was called back to interview with the man who would become my boss. I ultimately got the job. The position was to be an administrative assistant to the Director of East-West Studies at the Council on Foreign Relations. The Director's name was Michael Mandelbaum. That job ultimately launched me on my career path in the field of Russian area studies and Mr. Mandelbaum became my mentor.

As painful as the experience surrounding my failed first job was, there are two astonishing circumstances surrounding this event that are hard for me to view as mere coincidences. The first is the fact that if I had been fired just two days later, that job that launched me on my career path would have already been filled. The second is that between the time when I interviewed at the Council and the time I was offered the position, I traveled to Washington, D. C. for an interview with the National Security Agency. That interview was a grueling two-day process and by the end of the second day I was ready to go back to the hotel and sleep. However, a voice inside me told me to first call the employment agency. And how lucky it was that I did. They had been frantically calling everyone I had listed as a contact to try and reach me and tell me I had gotten the job. I shudder to think how things might have been different if I had not listened to that inner voice and had given into my desires to go back to the hotel and sleep.

The second turning point in my life was my ultimate choice of graduate schools. I had been working at the Council on Foreign Relations for almost three years, when the time came for me to think about pursuing graduate study. I had been living in New York City the whole time, had made many friends and even had a boyfriend. So, naturally, my inclination was to stay in New York, where I was happy, and stay, of course, with my boyfriend. Furthermore, the idea of moving to a new city and having to start all over was frightening, to say the least. I applied to both Columbia University's School of International Affairs in New York City and to The Johns Hopkins School of Advanced International Studies (SAIS) in Washington, D.C. I had visited SAIS during my sophomore year in college and had liked the school and its program very much. I had decided that this was where I would go to graduate school. However, that had been five years earlier. I was now living a great and exciting life in New York City and was quite content to stay put.

I applied to both schools and was accepted at both of them. At the time of my acceptance, neither school had offered me any financial aid. In fact, I had been told by a friend of mine who was attending SAIS at the time, not to expect any financial aid from that institution. So, I decided I would try to make it work financially through Columbia. Shortly after that, the financial aid office at SAIS called me and told me that they were prepared to offer me a substantial fellowship. Only eight fellowships were awarded that year to an incoming class of 100 to 120 students. There are those, of course, who will say that my ending up at SAIS had nothing to do with God's plans. "You got that fellowship because of your qualifications," I can hear them say. And I would counter, "You are correct. I *did* get that fellowship because of my qualifications. However, those same qualifications were on my application to Columbia. So why did I not receive any financial aid from Columbia, a far better-endowed university?"

With the offer of financial aid from SAIS and no offer of aid from Columbia, the writing was on the wall. Regardless of my desire to stay in New York, financial concerns were paramount. Still, I was determined to stay in New York. I made several attempts to make Columbia work out financially for me, to the point of obsession. I approached the problem from every conceivable angle, including the idea of going part-time and working at the school part-time, thereby getting a reduction in tuition. I was willing to put myself through a great deal of financial hardship, not to mention other hardships, to stay in New York City. Thankfully, cooler heads prevailed, namely those of my parents, and I headed to Washington, D. C. in August, 1989.

While the decision to attend SAIS was driven ultimately by financial reasons, I have come to believe it was God's plan for me to be in Washington, D. C. for a different reason. For starters, during the spring of my first year of graduate school, my former boss at the Council on Foreign Relations in New York City, Michael Mandelbaum, had moved to Washington, D. C. to accept the position of the Christian A. Herter Professor of American Foreign Policy and to be the Director of the American Foreign Policy program at SAIS, the very graduate school I was then attending. Both he and his wife, Anne, became close friends of my parents and provided endless emotional support to them during my three months at The George Washington University Medical Center (GWUMC). In addition, it was Anne who spearheaded a fundraising campaign to help offset my medical expenses. Although she could have done this from New York City, the fact that she and Michael were now based in Washington, D.C. and that Michael was a tenured professor at the very institution I was attending probably made it easier to accomplish. Later, with my father having passed away and my mother living 1500 miles away in Tulsa, Oklahoma, Anne and Michael Mandelbaum, became like second parents to me while I lived in Washington, D. C.

Secondly, my parents had both relatives and college friends in Washington, D. C., who opened their homes to them, giving them comfortable places to stay, where they could have their own space and not be in the way. With free room and board during the three and a half months they were in Washington, D.C., they were able to cut their expenses dramatically and be by my bedside as much as twelve hours a day. Finally, under the guidance of my father's law school friend, who lived in Arlington, Virginia, I started attending church and it was there that the process of my spiritual awakening began.

God's plans aside for placing me in Washington, D.C., I believe SAIS was the best possible graduate school for me to have attended, given what happened to me. The outpouring of financial, moral and emotional support that was shown to my parents and me amazes me to this day, seventeen years later. When I was at GWUMC for the first three months, my parents say I constantly received visits from friends, fellow students, even teachers. The Associate Dean of Students at SAIS, the late George L. Crowell, telephoned my parents on a weekly basis to check on my progress. He continued to do this even after I had been transferred to the Kaiser rehabilitation facility in Tulsa, Oklahoma. It was Dean Crowell, who personally went to bat for me against the insurance company to have a rehabilitation clause inserted into my contract after my surgery had gone awry, so that some of my rehabilitation expenses would be covered. Finally, upon returning to SAIS in 1992 after rehabilitation, the school administration went out of its way to make it physically and financially possible for me to complete my degree. They gave me extra time on my exams. The registrar scheduled my exams according to my needs and allowed me to turn in a term paper two semesters late, against school policy. I was also able to schedule my oral examination to give me enough time to prepare. Perhaps the school was just doing this because they were required to do so under the Americans With Disabilities Act. There is certainly no way to prove that I would not have had the same experience with the administration, the faculty and the students at Columbia. But, I tend to doubt it. Many of my friends, who attended Columbia, agree with this assessment. Columbia is a large university with a large bureaucracy. A single student can easily fall between the cracks.

A third turning point in my life was the events surrounding my discharge from GWUMC in Washington to Magee in Philadelphia. My parents had been trying to find a way for me to return to Tulsa for the continuation of my rehabilitation, because they wanted to get back to doctors whom they knew and trusted. The problem my parents faced was how to transport me there. I was unable to go by car. I was still on a stretcher. I could not go on an ordinary plane. I was still attached to tubes. It would have to be an air ambulance, specially equipped with medical machines, since taking a regular ambulance from Washington, D. C. to Tulsa would be impractical. An air ambulance was the only option, but that type of service was very expensive and more than my parents could afford.

My mother happened to speak on the telephone with a friend of hers in Tulsa about this predicament. That friend, in turn, called a friend of hers, Don Newman, whose son, Russell, was in the private medical aviation business. It happened that Russell Newman's older brother had attended high school with my sister, Carolyn. It also happened that the plane the Newmans owned was to be in Washington, D.C. at the same time as I was supposed to be released from the hospital. Mr. Newman offered the use of their plane to fly my mother, my father, and me back to Tulsa free of charge. All my parents had to pay for was the fuel required.

Everything had been arranged with St. Johns Medical Center in Tulsa and with my parents' internist, Dr. Stephen Gawey and the neurosurgeon on staff, Dr. R. Frank Tenney. The day before we were to leave Washington, D.C. for Tulsa, my father returned his and my mother's commercial airline tickets to the airline for a refund, while my mother and a friend of hers took my steamer trunk to the Greyhound bus terminal in northeast Washington, D. C. to be shipped to Tulsa. Everyone then proceeded to the hospital.

When my parents arrived at GWUMC, the social worker there told them that someone at St. Johns in Tulsa had called to say that the hospital would not admit me as I was so close to starting the rehabilitation phase of my recovery and there was no rehabilitative type of coverage in my insurance policy from the school. Why would there be? What student insurance policy would anticipate that a twenty-six year-old student is going to need catastrophic coverage? Needless to say, my parents were devastated.

After numerous calls to physicians in Tulsa to see if anything could be worked out, my parents went to see George Crowell, the Associate Dean of Students at SAIS. He, in turn, put them in touch with the school's insurance broker, Sam Shriver. As you may recall, it was at that point that Mr. Shriver worked with the school and went to bat for me with Blue Cross/Blue Shield and got the ball rolling on getting a rehabilitation clause inserted in my student policy so that I could get into a rehabilitation facility. I was evaluated by several different social workers from various rehabilitation hospitals in Washington, D.C, as well as a representative from Magee. My parents were asked to visit Magee. The day after that visit, they were told that Blue Cross/Blue Shield had authorized treatment for me at Magee. So I went by ambulance to Magee and my parents followed behind the ambulance in their car.

The morning after they arrived, my parents met with the social worker at Magee. She advised my parents to go home to Tulsa after the staff at Magee had met with them so that my parents could get their affairs in order and then return. The staff at Magee wanted to evaluate me without parental distractions and my parents, after all, had been away for three months longer than they had originally expected.

So, everything was set, except for one thing. How would my parents get back to Tulsa? My father had turned in their return tickets to Tulsa the day before, not knowing that the original plan for him, my mother, and me to return to Tulsa on an air ambulance would fall through, because of St. John's refusal to accept me. Last-minute one-way fares were prohibitively expensive. Uncertain how they could afford to return to Tulsa, my parents headed back to Virginia where they had been staying with friends during my hospitalization in Washington, D. C., stopping off at a neighborhood grocery store to pick up some groceries. As my mother started to unload the groceries from the paper bag, she read an advertisement on the side of the bag about a promotional offer that Mid West Airlines was running, stating that if a customer purchased groceries of a certain value, the

Airline would give the customer a free air ticket. By chance, my mother had purchased exactly enough for two tickets. With glee she turned to my father and exclaimed, "Honey, here's how we're getting home!"

Again, I have asked myself, were these events nothing but a series of coincidences? Or were they all part of a divine plan to place me where I needed to be to receive the therapy I needed? As I wrote earlier, it is Magee that deserves the lion's share of the credit for truly bringing me along and for making it possible for me to walk and to have full use of my left arm.

I could list countless moments when I have come to believe God intervened to place me at the right place at the right time to get the help I needed, but I will mention only three more. The first is the process by which I found my physical therapist in Washington, D. C.

I had been without physical therapy for almost two years since returning to graduate school and my leg and foot were beginning to show the results of no longer being in physical therapy. Indeed, my balance and my problem with severe fatigue were getting worse with time. There happened to be an older lady living next door to me in the building where I lived. I noticed that a young woman would come to her door about once a week for a couple of hours and then leave. Being the curious sort, I stopped and asked her if she was a physical therapist. "No," she replied. "I'm an occupational therapist." "Why? Do you need a physical therapist?"

I explained my situation and she gave me the name of a physical therapist, Susan Ryerson, with whom she had worked. She told me that Susan was known for "thinking outside the box" and not approaching every situation with the standard, textbook remedies.

"Just the woman for me," I thought. And so I went to see her shortly thereafter. That meeting proved to be instrumental to my further recovery, because, true to her reputation, Susan Ryerson did not approach every case with the same tried and true methods. She was innovative. I met her for the first time in 1994 and continued in treatment with her until I left Washington, D. C. in 2005. Susan's open minded approach to therapy resulted in my moving out of a large, clunky brace to a small, lightweight molded plastic brace that fit inside my shoe. A person who does not wear a brace might find it difficult to understand what a huge psychological impact that had on me. No longer did I have the "disabled" label for all to see, because the brace was so small, you didn't really notice it unless I pointed it out. The smaller brace also enabled me to wear regular flat-soled shoes rather than always having to walk in tennis shoes. I could also wear shoes that were close to my normal size, 6 ½, rather than a size 8 for the left foot so that it would fit over the brace and a size 6 ½ for my right foot.

Susan also introduced me to a hand-held functional electrical simulation device manufactured by Empi and worked with me to get insurance coverage to pay for it. This device uses electrical stimulation to try to reestablish contact with a muscle and to provide sensory input back to the part of the brain that controls the muscle. The therapist locates the muscle that controls the part of the foot, finger or arm that needs strengthening and places electrodes on that muscle.

SEARCHING FOR THE OPEN DOOR

Even after my departure from Washington, D. C. in 2005, I have remained in touch with Susan. It is through her that I became aware of two new electrical stimulation devices coming out on the market: the Bioness L300 and the WalkAid from Hanger. These two devices incorporate sophisticated software that allows stimulation of the muscle during the appropriate phase of walking.

Many might think it a lucky series of breaks that I had the curiosity to speak with my neighbor's occupational therapist, a total stranger, and she referred me to Susan Ryerson and that I decided to begin physical therapy with Susan based on her recommendation. However, there are some 261 physical therapists that operate in and around the greater Washington, D. C. area. I have been to several of them during my thirteen years in Washington, D. C. All of them approached the problem of treating my disability using the same conventional methods they had learned in school. I had not progressed with any of them. I have often asked myself, "What are the chances that I just happened to live next door to someone who was getting occupational therapy and *that* occupational therapist, in turn, referred me to a physical therapist, who *could* help me?" Some may say coincidence or just dumb luck. I say divine intervention.

The events surrounding my father's death have served to further reinforce my belief in a greater being in control of the universe. The date was April 30, 1999, a Friday. I was working at the U.S. Trade and Development Agency in Washington, D. C. and had come back to my apartment briefly to pack for a conference I was about to attend in New York City. The phone rang just as I entered my apartment. It was my mother. She told me that my father, who had been admitted to the hospital a week earlier for complications surrounding lymphoma cancer, had just gone into cardiac arrest. The doctors had succeeded in reviving him, but he was in a coma. My mother was calling all three of her daughters so that we could make travel arrangements to come home to Tulsa that night. The doctors had told my mother that my father did not have long to live.

I made my plane reservations, but because I was traveling to Tulsa, I would have to change planes either in St. Louis, Dallas, or Chicago. I chose TWA, which had the best connections but I still would not arrive in Tulsa until close to 9:00 P.M. I felt that it was likely that I would never see my father alive again.

God put two angels in my path that day. The first was the lady who walked me with my baggage to the plane. As I mentioned in Chapter Two, when I get emotional, my leg doesn't function properly. I basically can't walk. And I definitely was emotional that day. I would never have physically been able to get to the gate if that lady hadn't been standing next to me at the ticket counter.

The second angel in my path that day came in the guise of a young man, who wheeled me to my connecting flight in St. Louis. Our plane that left Washington, D.C. had arrived in St. Louis, forty-five minutes ahead of time; in time to catch an earlier connection to Tulsa. The pilot explained that we had caught a huge tailwind. This was truly incredible, because tailwinds ordinarily travel from west to east, not from east to west. The other extraordinary part of this trip was that there was a gate available for us, even though we were forty-five minutes early.

The plane landed in St. Louis and we arrived at the gate. I explained the situation – that I was attempting to catch an earlier flight to Tulsa and that my father was dying - to the man awaiting the plane's arrival with a wheelchair for me and we rushed off. Upon arriving at the transfer gate, he left me for a moment to talk to the agent at the counter. I saw the agent shake his head. The plane was full. There were no seats. At this point, I began sobbing. I think it was something about seeing me wracked with powerful emotion, a heaving body in a wheelchair that moved the counter attendant's heart. "Come here," he said. "I'll get you on this plane, even if I have to put you in first class."

And so he did. I arrived at Tulsa International Airport at 6:30 P.M. rushed over to St. John Medical Center's Intensive Care Unit (ICU) and stood by my father's bedside, just as he opened his eyes. My father faded in and out of consciousness for the next day and a half, giving my sisters the chance to arrive and for the family as a whole to say goodbye. In the end, his body was overwhelmed with infection and the complications from his diabetes and his chemotherapy. We made the decision to remove his life support and all four of us – my mother, my two sisters and I – sat quietly by his bedside as life slowly left his body. They say that a person's soul animates his whole body. That statement perfectly describes the scene at my father's deathbed. My father was a great man. He was the first love of my life, just as I was the apple of his eye. His spirit seemed to leave his body quickly. In the end, all that was left of my father was a shell. My father was gone. To this day, I am grateful that I was given the chance to say goodbye. At his memorial service, I told people that I could not imagine living life without my father. Now, I know I must go on living, if only because my father continues to live inside of me.

The circumstances through which I met my husband is the final example I will present. I was one week shy of my thirty-seventh birthday and living alone in Washington, D.C. Although I had dated quite a bit, no relationship had worked out for me and I had a good idea why. First, Washington, D. C. is a magnet for political insiders and people who want to be political movers and shakers. I did not fit the stereotype of the political wife or anyone's idea of a political partner. I was disabled. I was also very outspoken, undiplomatically so. And, I wasn't getting any younger as the saying goes. I had pretty much given up on getting married and was finally at peace with my life, as mundane and humdrum as it was. And then along came my future husband.

I met Steve through my sister, Carolyn, who lives in Fort Lauderdale, where my husband and I now live. Steve was forty-three at the time and, like me, had pretty much given up on getting married. Steve was told about me through a mutual friend of his and Carolyn's and he decided to call me. According to him, his first impression of me was that I sounded like a stuck up East Coast person and, after speaking with me for a few minutes, he hung up the phone, determined never to call me again. Then came Thanksgiving, 2000. I decided at the last minute to go with my girl friend to Florida and spend Thanksgiving with my sister, not realizing that she already had plans to fly to Los Angeles to be with her husband. I had already bought a round trip plane ticket to

Fort Lauderdale and I was thus faced with the prospect of spending Thanksgiving in a city that I didn't know at all.

It was then that Rebecca intervened. Rebecca was the friend, who knew both Carolyn and Steve. Playing the sympathy card, Rebecca convinced Steve to give me a second chance and invite me and my friend to Thanksgiving dinner. A co-worker of his asked him what he was doing for Thanksgiving. Steve told her, in a rather disgusted tone of voice, that, unfortunately, he had gotten roped into entertaining for Thanksgiving this girl whose sister had reneged on an invitation to spend the holiday together. He was planning to spend the day with me and then leave me and my girl friend and get together with a friend of *his,* who was also coming to town for the holiday.

"I thought you were going snowmobiling in Colorado?" his co-worker said.

"Well, apparently there is no snow, so my buddy is coming here."

And with that he left the office. Four days later, upon his return to the office, that same co-worker asked him how his Thanksgiving holiday had gone and how was the girl.

"I think I just met my future wife," was his reply.

Our friends ask me to retell this story all the time. I tell them, "Steve and I tried really hard not to meet each other." I was scared. After all, I was almost 37 and had orchestrated quite a nice life for myself. In addition, at 37, I was unsure whether I could adapt to the intrusion of another human being into my ordered life. I was also being continually warned by my sister that Steve was not a believer and since I *was* a believer, this meant that our union would not be in accordance with Biblical principles, the principle of being "equally yoked." I ignored those warnings, obviously. I decided that being "unequally yoked" does not preclude a happy marriage.

Steve and I have now been happily married for over five years and I love him more today than the day I married him. He is perfect for me and we mesh together perfectly. His strengths are my weaknesses and the reverse is also true. Like me, he has a disability and that is a strong bond. Both of us know what it takes to make it in this world with a disability and both of us understand the discrimination and obstacles that are constantly put in our path because of our disabilities. Through him, I have found the courage to push the envelope and push myself beyond what I thought I could do. Since our marriage, I have begun driving again. I am also no longer confined to the six block radius that was my life in Washington, D. C. I have picked up and moved 1,000 miles to a completely new life in a new state whose culture and lifestyle is very different from anything I've known before.

Sharing life with a man of my husband's adventurous spirit and zest for living has been a constant source of joy for me. Steve's love of life is contagious. His ingenuity, his imagination and his spirit are only a few of the qualities of his that inspire me every day of my life. After the blessing of being born to loving parents, the greatest blessing of my life has been my marriage to this caring, brilliant and loving man.

Moving to Florida has been a challenge, and I have not yet adjusted fully to the change, but I know it is only a matter of time. Everything is in God's time. I truly believe that God intended for Steve and me to meet at that very time in our lives. If we had met any earlier, neither of us would have been in a position, emotionally or in terms of our maturity, to get married. At a different time in our lives, having taken different paths, it is likely that neither of us would have been receptive even to meeting the other. I had grandiose plans of working and traveling abroad. Many of my college and graduate school class-mates are now pursuing the very goals that had been mine. Many of them find their work, their travels and their lives fulfilling. I have found a life that is equally fulfilling. And so, yet again, God has taken what at first seemed like a tragedy and brought forth something more beautiful than anything I ever could have imagined - love.

ABOUT THE AUTHOR

Cynthia Paddock Doroghazi was on her way to what she thought would be a flourishing career as a specialist in Russian-area studies when she suffered a traumatic brain injury that left her paralyzed on her left side and in a coma. The injury changed the course of her life. Her B.A. in Russian Studies from Amherst College and her M.A. in International Relations from the Johns Hopkins School of Advanced International Studies suddenly seemed irrelevant. No longer able to pursue her intended career in Russian Studies as a Russian area specialist or diplomat, Cynthia began to pursue other talents and discovered that she had very strong organizational skills, which has led to a promising career in event planning. She also found she excelled in public speaking. In fact, she became a District 36, Toastmasters' International Speech contest champion in 1999. Her plan is to use this talent to become a motivational speaker on behalf of people with disabilities. Born in Tulsa, Oklahoma, Cynthia lived for fourteen years in Washington, D. C. before moving to Ft. Lauderdale, FL where she currently resides. She is married to Stephen Doroghazi, a blind attorney, who himself has overcome obstacles in pursuit of success, and who became a genuine source of strength for her completing this book.